# The Craft
# of Teaching About Families:
# Strategies and Tools

*The Craft of Teaching About Families: Strategies and Tools* has been previously published as *Marriage & Family Review*, Volume 38, Numbers 2/3/4 2005.

> **Monographic Separates from *Marriage & Family Review***
>
> For additional information on these and other Haworth Press titles, including descriptions, tables of contents, reviews, and prices, use the QuickSearch catalog at http://www.HaworthPress.com.

*The Craft of Teaching About Families: Strategies and Tools,* edited by Debra L. Berke and Steven K. Wisensale (Vol. 38, No. 2/3/4, 2005). *"A superb resource for all who teach about families, this collection offers concrete examples focusing on how to teach family policy, research, and clinical techniques effectively. The breadth of coverage is impressive. . . . This book offers an exciting array of ideas and suggestions–all grounded and tested in real classrooms with real students. . . . Should be read cover-to-cover by all of us concerned with teaching the next generation of family scholars, advocates, and practitioners."* (Eileen Trzcinski, PhD, Professor and Director of Social Work, Wayne State University)

*Challenges of Aging on U.S. Families: Policy and Practice Implications,* edited by Richard K. Caputo, PhD (Vol. 37, No. 1/2, 2005). *Examines the policy and practical implications of the aging United States population, the changes within the family structure, caregiving by various family members, and the overall economic impact.*

*Parent-Youth Relations: Cultural and Cross-Cultural Perspectives,* edited by Gary W. Peterson, Suzanne K. Steinmetz, and Stephan M. Wilson (Vol. 35, No. 3/4, 2003; Vol. 36, No. 1/2/3/4, 2004). *A comprehensive examination of how culture interconnects with parent-child relationships.*

*Emotions and the Family,* edited by Richard A. Fabes, PhD (Vol. 34, No. 1/2/3/4 2002). *"An exciting collection. The contributors insightfully unfold the nature of emotions as relational processes in marriage and parenting, and illuminate how emotional communication, competence, and regulation color family life. Chapters on siblings, stepfamilies, economic stress, and family therapy add richness to the collective portrayal of how emotions infuse marital and parent-child relationships. Scholars of marital and family life will find this a valuable resource."* (Ross A. Thompson, PhD, Carl A. Happold Distinguished Professor of Psychology, University of Nebraska)

*Gene-Environment Processes in Social Behaviors and Relationships,* edited by Kirby Deater-Deckard, PhD, and Stephen A. Petrill, PhD (Vol. 33, No. 1/2/3, 2002). *"During recent years there have been somewhat fruitless battles on whether family influences or peer influences are more important in children's psychological development. This book is both innovative and helpful in seeking to bring the two sets of influences together through a range of studies using twin, adoptee, and stepfamily designs to assess how genetic and environmental influences may work together in bringing about individual differences in children's emotions, behavior and especially social relationships. The different research approaches provide some new ways of thinking about, and investigating, how interpersonal relationships develop and have their effects."* (Michael Rutter, MD, FRS, Professor of Developmental Psychopathology, Institute of Psychiatry, King's College, London)

*Pioneering Paths in the Study of Families: The Lives and Careers of Family Scholars,* edited by Suzanne K. Steinmetz, PhD, MSW, and Gary W. Peterson, PhD (Vol. 30, No. 3, 2000; Vol. 30, No. 4, 2001; Vol. 31, No. 1/2/3/4, 2001; Vol. 32, No. 1/2, 2001). *The fascinating autobiographies of 40 leading scholars in sociology, family studies, psychology, and child development.*

*FATHERHOOD: Research, Interventions and Policies,* edited by H. Elizabeth Peters, PhD, Gary W. Peterson, PhD, Suzanne K. Steinmetz, PhD, MSW, and Randal D. Day, PhD (Vol. 29, No. 2/3/4, 2000). *Brings together the latest facts to help researchers explore the father-child relationship and determine what factors lead fathers to be more or less involved in the lives of their children, including human social behavior, not living with a child, being denied visiting privileges, and social norms regarding gender differences versus work responsibilities.*

*Concepts and Definitions of Family for the 21st Century,* edited by Barbara H. Settles, PhD, Suzanne K. Steinmetz, PhD, MSW, Gary W. Peterson, PhD, and Marvin B. Sussman, PhD (Vol. 28, No. 3/4, 1999). *Views family from a U.S. perspective and from many different cultures and societies. The controversial question "What is family?" is thoroughly examined as it has become an increasingly important social policy concern in recent years as the traditional family has changed.*

*The Role of the Hospitality Industry in the Lives of Individuals and Families,* edited by Pamela R. Cummings, PhD, Francis A. Kwansa, PhD, and Marvin B. Sussman, PhD (Vol. 28, No. 1/2, 1998). *"A must for human resource directors and hospitality educators." (Dr. Lynn Huffman, Director, Restaurant, Hotel, and Institutional Management, Texas Tech University, Lubbock, Texas)*

*Stepfamilies: History, Research, and Policy,* edited by Irene Levin, PhD, and Marvin B. Sussman, PhD (Vol. 26, No. 1/2/3/4, 1997). *"A wide range of individually valuable and stimulating chapters that form a wonderfully rich menu from which readers of many different kinds will find exciting and satisfying selections." (Jon Bernardes, PhD, Principal Lecturer in Sociology, University of Wolverhampton, Castle View Dudley, United Kingdom)*

*Families and Adoption,* edited by Harriet E. Gross, PhD, and Marvin B. Sussman, PhD (Vol. 25, No. 1/2/3/4, 1997). *"Written in a lucid and easy-to-read style, this volume will make an invaluable contribution to the adoption literature." (Paul Sachdev, PhD, Professor, School of Social Work, Memorial University of Newfoundland, St. John's, Newfoundland, Canada)*

*The Methods and Methodologies of Qualitative Family Research,* edited by Jane F. Gilgun, PhD, LICSW, and Marvin B. Sussman, PhD (Vol 24, No. 1/2/3/4, 1997). *"An authoritative look at the usefulness of qualitative research methods to the family scholar." (Family Relations)*

*Intercultural Variation in Family Research and Theory: Implications for Cross-National Studies,* Volumes I and II, edited by Marvin B. Sussman, PhD, and Roma S. Hanks, PhD (Vol. 22, No. 1/2/3/4, and Vol. 23, No. 1/2/3/4, 1997). *Documents the development of family research in theory in societies around the world and inspires continued cross-national collaboration on current research topics.*

*Families and Law,* edited by Lisa J. McIntyre, PhD, and Marvin B. Sussman, PhD (Vol. 21, No. 3/4, 1995). *With this new volume, family practitioners and scholars can begin to increase the family's position in relation to the law and legal system.*

*Exemplary Social Intervention Programs for Members and Their Families,* edited by David Guttmann, DSW, and Marvin B. Sussman, PhD (Vol. 21, No. 1/2, 1995). *An eye-opening look at organizations and individuals who have created model family programs that bring desired results.*

*Single Parent Families: Diversity, Myths and Realities,* edited by Shirley M. H. Hanson, RN, PhD, Marsha L. Heims, RN, EdD, Doris J. Julian, RN, EdD, and Marvin B. Sussman, PhD (Vol. 20, No. 1/2/3/4, 1994). *"Remarkable! . . . A significant work and is important reading for multidisciplinary family professionals including sociologists, educators, health care professionals, and policymakers." (Maureen Leahey, RN, PhD, Director, Outpatient Mental Health Program, Director, Family Therapy Training Program, Calgary District Hospital Group)*

*Families on the Move: Immigration, Migration, and Mobility,* edited by Barbara H. Settles, PhD, Daniel E. Hanks III, MS, and Marvin B. Sussman, PhD (Vol 19, No 1/2/3/4, 1993). *Examines the current research on family mobility, migration, and immigration and discovers new directions for understanding the relationship between mobility and family life.*

*American Families and the Future: Analyses of Possible Destinies,* edited by Barbara H. Settles, PhD, Roma S. Hanks, PhD, and Marvin B. Sussman, PhD (Vol. 18, No. 3/4, 1993). *This book discusses a variety of issues that face and will continue to face families in coming years and describes various strategies families can use in their decision-making processes.*

*Publishing in Journals on the Family: Essays on Publishing,* edited by Roma S. Hanks, PhD, Linda Matocha, PhD, RN, and Marvin B. Sussman, PhD (Vol. 18, No. 1/2, 1993). *This helpful book contains varied perspectives from scholars at different career stages and from editors of major publication outlets, providing readers with important information necessary to help them systematically plan a productive scholarly career.*

*Publishing in Journals on the Family: A Survey and Guide for Scholars, Practitioners, and Students,* edited by Roma S. Hanks, PhD, Linda Matocha, PhD, RN, and Marvin B. Sussman, PhD (Vol. 17, No. 3/4, 1992). *"Comprehensive. . . . Includes listings for some 200 social science journals whose editors have expressed an interest in publishing empirical research and theoretical articles about the family." (Reference & Research Book News)*

# The Craft of Teaching About Families: Strategies and Tools

Debra L. Berke
Steven K. Wisensale
Editors

*The Craft of Teaching About Families: Strategies and Tools* has been previously published as *Marriage & Family Review*, Volume 38, Numbers 2/3/4 2005.

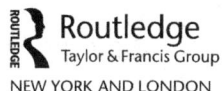

NEW YORK AND LONDON

First Published by

The Haworth Press, Inc., 10 Alice Street, Binghamton, NY 13904-1580 USA

This edition published 2011 by Routledge
711 Third Avenue, New York, NY 10017
2 Park Square, Milton Park, Abingdon, Oxon, OX14 4RN

*The Craft of Teaching About Families: Strategies and Tools* has been previously published as *Marriage & Family Review*, Volume 38, Numbers 2/3/4 2005.

© 2005 by The Haworth Press, Inc. All rights reserved. No part of this work may be reproduced or utilized in any form or by any means, electronic or mechanical, including photocopying, microfilm and recording, or by any information storage and retrieval system, without permission in writing from the publisher.

The development, preparation, and publication of this work has been undertaken with great care. However, the publisher, employees, editors, and agents of The Haworth Press and all imprints of The Haworth Press, Inc., including The Haworth Medical Press® and Pharmaceutical Products Press®, are not responsible for any errors contained herein or for consequences that may ensue from use of materials or information contained in this work. With regard to case studies, identities and circumstances of individuals discussed herein have been changed to protect confidentiality. Any resemblance to actual persons, living or dead, is entirely coincidental.

The Haworth Press is committed to the dissemination of ideas and information according to the highest standards of intellectual freedom and the free exchange of ideas. Statements made and opinions expressed in this publication do not necessarily reflect the views of the Publisher, Directors, management, or staff of The Haworth Press, Inc., or an endorsement by them.

Cover design by Kerry E. Mack

**Library of Congress Cataloging-in-Publication Data**

The craft of teaching about families : strategies and tools / Debra L. Berke, Steven K. Wisensale, editors.
    p. cm.
    "Co-published simultaneously as Marriage & family review, volume 38, numbers 2/3/4 2005."
    Includes bibliographical references and index.
    ISBN-13: 978-0-7890-3249-2 (hard cover : alk. paper)
    ISBN-10: 0-7890-3249-X (hard cover : alk. paper)
    ISBN-13: 978-0-7890-3250-8 (soft cover : alk. paper)
    ISBN-10: 0-7890-3250-3 (soft cover : alk. paper)
    1. Family–Study and teaching. 2. Family life education. 3. Family policy–Study and teaching.
I. Berke, Debra L. II. Wisensale, Steven K., 1945- III. Marriage & family review.

HQ10.C69 2006
306.85071′1–dc22

2006024794

# The Craft of Teaching About Families: Strategies and Tools

## CONTENTS

### TEACHING FAMILY LAW AND FAMILY POLICY

Editors' Comments     3
   *Debra L. Berke*
   *Steven K. Wisensale*

Writing *Amicus Curiae* and Policy Briefs:
   A Pedagogical Approach to Teaching Family Law and Policy     7
   *Preston A. Britner*
   *Lily T. Alpert*

Family Law and Foster Care: Cooperative Research Teams     25
   *Tammy L. Henderson*
   *Lenore McWey*

An Exploratory Examination of Students' Family Policy Beliefs     47
   *Randy Leite*
   *Ruben P. Viramontez Anguiano*

Teaching Family Policy: Advocacy Skills Education     63
   *Elaine A. Anderson*
   *Bonnie Braun*
   *Susan K. Walker*

Involving Marginalized Families in Shaping Policies:
   Roles for Cooperative Extension     79
   *Kimberly Greder*
   *Jeanne Warning*

## FAMILY DYNAMICS

Fathers and Daughters: A Needed Course in Family Studies    101
*Linda Nielsen*

Service-Learning in Parenting Education:
   Insights from Students and Parent Participants    115
*Rhonda A. Richardson*
*Audrey Kraynak*
*Maureen Blankemeyer*
*Kathleen A. Walker*

Teaching About International Families Across the United States    133
*Mihaela Robila*
*Alan C. Taylor*

International Families in Cross-Cultural Perspective:
   A Family Strengths Approach    147
*Nilufer P. Medora*

An Integrative Approach to Teaching Family Resource
   Management    165
*Jeanne M. Hilton*
*Karen Kopera-Frye*

## TEACHING TECHNIQUES IN FAMILY STUDIES

Creating Families: A Teaching Technique
   for Clinical Training Through Role-Playing    185
*Scott Browning*
*Jeanne S. Collins*
*Bryan Nelson*

Small-Group Learning and Hypothetical Families
   in a Large Introductory Course    205
*Tanya Koropeckyj-Cox*
*Colleen Cain*
*Justin Coran*

Psychological Abuse in Family Studies: A Psychoeducational
   and Preventive Approach     225
   *James M. O'Neil*
   *Stephen A. Anderson*
   *Preston A. Britner*
   *Irene Q. Brown*
   *Kathleen Holgerson*
   *Ronald P. Rohner*

Process Evaluation of Teaching Forgiveness in a Workshop
   and Classroom Setting     243
   *James M. O'Neil*
   *Diane Davison*
   *Matthew S. Mutchler*
   *Jennifer Trachtenberg*

The Impact of Service-Learning on Student Development:
   Students' Reflections in a Family Diversity Course     263
   *Michelle L. Toews*
   *Jennifer M. Cerny*

Index     281

## ABOUT THE EDITORS

**Debra L. Berke, PhD, CFLE,** is Associate Professor of Family Science and Women's Studies in the Department of Human Development and Family Science at Messiah College. She also directs the Gender Studies Project at Messiah College. Her research and teaching interests include work and family, family policy, human sexuality and teaching methodologies.

**Steven K. Wisensale, PhD,** is Professor of Public Policy in the School of Family Studies at the University of Connecticut. His research and teaching interests are in social welfare policy with a particular focus on family policy. He has published extensively in major professional journals and is the author of *Family Leave Policy: The Political Economy of Work and Family in America* (M.E. Sharpe, 2001).

# *TEACHING FAMILY LAW AND FAMILY POLICY*

# Editors' Comments

Debra L. Berke
Steven K. Wisensale

Once on the back burner of university curricula, Family Studies continues to gain greater recognition and respect as a discipline. Clearly, this is a reflection of developments in society as a whole, with stories about controversial family issues surfacing almost daily in the national media and greater attention being devoted to family matters by legislatures and courts with each passing year. What was once personal and private has become part of public debates and political campaigns. It is within this context that instructors must teach and students must learn about the complexities of today's families.

However, teaching is an occupation practiced in private. "Professors . . . walk into the classroom and close the door–figuratively and literally–on the daunting task of teaching. When we emerge we rarely talk with each other about what we have done, or need to do" (Palmer, 1993, p. 8). Shulman (1993) calls this "pedagogical solitude." These articles in this collection make the private public through their scholarship. Each article exemplifies the scholarship of teaching and learning (Boyer, 1990) as they reflect on teaching about families.

As presented in this stimulating collection of papers, there are a variety of course designs and teaching strategies that can be employed to address the complexities of family life in the twenty-first century. Aware of the challenges that students will face as they leave the campus for the real world, instructors strive to provide their charges with not only a solid knowledge base in family science, but to arm them with the appropriate skills they need to solve problems that may not yet exist. Therefore, it is only fitting that the topics covered in these papers include family law and policy, advocacy, parenting skills, international families, and diversity, among others.

The collection will be presented in three subsequent issues of *Marriage & Family Review*. With respect to the first set of articles, the focus is on family law and policy. Britner and Alpert's excellent article on building writing skills through the preparation of court briefs and policy memos is complemented by Henderson and McWey's innovative approach to teaching family law through the use of cooperative learning research teams. The Leite and Viramontez Anguiano paper reminds us that we should devote some time early in our policy courses to gauging our students' knowledge and perspectives on various issues. And while the Anderson, Braun and Walker article focuses on advocacy skills, the Greder and Warning paper carries the concept a step further through the use of simulations and role-playing that are applied to a community setting.

While the first set of papers explores skill-building strategies, advocacy techniques, and policy issues from a macro perspective, the second set of articles, to appear in a subsequent issue, concentrates primarily on family dynamics. For example, Linda Nielsen argues strongly for a course on fathers and daughters and then goes on to offer an excellent blueprint for those who wish to follow her recommendation. In Richardson et al.'s work we learn how to convert a course in parenting education into a service learning activity. Robila and Taylor's paper on international families is complemented by Medora's work on the importance of creating a cross-cultural perspective when teaching about families. And finally, Hilton and Kopera-Frye remind us of the importance of family resource management as a subject field and not only argue for its inclusion in the curriculum, but provide us with a model for doing so.

The final set of papers, also in a subsequent issue, serves as an excellent resource for teaching techniques in clinical settings, small groups, and special workshops. Browning, Nelson and Collins recommend the use of a role-playing technique as part of clinical training. Koropeckyj-Cox, Cain, and Coran discuss the value of using hypothetical families in small group discussions in a large introductory course. O'Neil et al. provide us with two excellent articles. One concerns teaching about psychological abuse in families, with a particular emphasis on prevention. The other explores a process evaluation for a workshop on forgiveness. And, for our final paper in this collection, Toews and Cerny examine the impact of service learning on student development in a family diversity course.

As we move forward in teaching family studies, we need to remind ourselves that there are few venues, other than a published collection of papers like this one, where we can exchange teaching strategies and seek advice from each other. Most professional conferences tend to be biased toward research presentations, not panels on teaching family studies. Currently there is only one organization, the Family Science Association, which strives to enhance the teaching of family science; for more information about the Family Science Association, see their website: http://wcuvax1.wcu.edu/~lroberts/FSA.html. The National Council on Family Relations has a Section whose mission is to expand, strengthen, and enhance family science as a scholarship discipline–the Family Science Section–that sponsors sessions on teaching but it is one of the smallest Sections of NCFR. Therefore, we need to think of better ways to communicate with each other and expand our ways of sharing our knowledge and pedagogical skills. Perhaps within our respective professional organizations we can start a new section or special interest group on teaching about families or work to expand groups which already exist. Or, perhaps we can create a listserv that is devoted exclusively to teaching courses in family studies. A more ambitious project of course would entail the establishment of a Web site where ideas could be exchanged and discussed, syllabi could be made available, and reports and papers could be posted. Thus, instead of viewing this collection as a final project, we should instead look upon it as a reaffirmation of the importance of teaching for those of us who care about teaching.

## REFERENCES

Boyer, E. L. (1990). *Scholarship reconsidered: Priorities of the professoriate.* Princeton, NJ: The Carnegie Foundation for the Advancement of Teaching.

Palmer, P. (1993). Good talk about good teaching: Improving teaching through conversation and community. *Change, 25*, 8-13.

Shulman, L. (1993). Teaching as community property: Putting an end to pedagogical solitude. *Change, 25*, 6-7.

# Writing *Amicus Curiae* and Policy Briefs: A Pedagogical Approach to Teaching Family Law and Policy

Preston A. Britner
Lily T. Alpert

**ABSTRACT.** In this article, we make an argument for the importance of policy education for marriage and family students as a way of promoting critical thinking and engagement in science translation or advocacy. Several relevant active pedagogical approaches to teaching about law/policy are reviewed. We then describe the objectives and assignments from a class on Child Welfare, Law, and Social Policy, including written policy briefs and *amicus curiae* (friend of the court) legal briefs, and subsequent oral presentations. Student feedback is presented from eight classes with undergraduates and graduate students over a five-year period. We end with some conclusions about the approach. *[Article copies available for a fee from The Haworth Document Delivery Service: 1-800-HAWORTH. E-mail address: <docdelivery@haworthpress.com> Website: <http://www.HaworthPress.com> © 2005 by The Haworth Press, Inc. All rights reserved.]*

**KEYWORDS.** *Amicus curiae* brief, family law, family policy, family studies, pedagogy, policy brief, student feedback

---

Preston A. Britner and Lily T. Alpert are affiliated with the University of Connecticut.
Address correspondence to: Preston A. Britner, PhD, School of Family Studies, University of Connecticut, U-2058, Storrs, CT 06269-2058 USA (E-mail: britner@uconn.edu).
The first author teaches the courses described in the paper; the second author took the graduate version of the course and lived to tell about it.

## INTRODUCTION

Courses in policy and law are important for students studying marriage and family relations because they contribute to students' awareness of the interplay between family life and non-family aspects of the society. Scholars note that one major goal of a family policy/law course is to give students an understanding of "the intersection of the law and family development and how political, sociocultural, and economic processes influence the development and implementation of family law" (Henderson & Martin, 2002, p. 358). Students must understand how policies and laws affect families (e.g., Bogenschneider, 2002; Rickel & Becker, 1997) and how research can affect laws and policies (e.g., Bogenschneider, 2002; Melton, 1987). They must understand the policy or legal arena before designing their studies, in order to design studies that address the relevant legal/policy questions (Reppucci & Aber, 1987).

Several recurrent themes appear in the discussion of essential components of policy courses. Many authors agree that the goals of such courses should include an increase in students' critical thinking skills, full engagement of students in the course content, and an increase in students' knowledge of course material (Endersby & Webber, 1995; Keller, Whittaker, & Burke, 2001), as well as an acknowledgement of the contextual nature of public policy (Anderson & Skinner, 1995; Boyd, 1989; Brunner, 1997). In addition, researchers agree that policy courses should go beyond the delivery of course material. A successful policy course prepares its students to be educated and active consumers of public policy information. Furthermore, students should emerge from such a course better able to participate in the policymaking process (Henderson & Martin, 2002; Rocha & Johnson, 1997).

Describing the goals of a Master of Public Administration (MPA) program at Columbia, Cohen, Eimicke, and Ukeles (1995) write: "In our view, the goal of the public policy program is to create public sector problem solvers: people who are agile, flexible, politically astute, modest, and humble in the face of greater experience" (pp. 620-621). Many of the same attributes and skills seem to pop up on lists of desirable characteristics across a variety of social and human service fields.

## RELEVANT PEDAGOGICAL APPROACHES

This paper fits with recent attempts to bridge teaching with scholarship (Huber, 2004). We briefly review some of the relevant pedagogical approaches that have informed the development of the course.

## Active Learning and Critical Thinking

The literature suggests that a multifaceted, "hands-on" kind of curriculum (as opposed to the passive lecture and exam approach) is the most effective way to create a course on public policy (Anderson & Skinner, 1995). These curricula take the policymaking process from the abstract to the practical, offering students the opportunity to learn by doing. Instructors have developed creative ways to incorporate this active learning style into their classes.

A variety of active learning approaches have been attempted by instructors. Debating has been suggested as an effective method in family policy classrooms (Anderson & Skinner, 1995). Keller and colleagues (2001) describe a child and family policy course for social work masters' students in which policy debating was the students' central project. Students were assigned to opposing sides of debates on various child welfare topics. Teams of students prepared their cases and debates were conducted in a professional way, allowing fixed amounts of time for statements, rebuttals and questions. The authors found that the exercise was effective in helping students identify their values, analyze competing positions, and advocate for their point.

Rocha and Johnson (1997) use other active learning styles in their social work course. For one assignment, students combined their family policy knowledge with policy practice skills to produce a "written communiqué"–an op/ed piece or legislative proposal. In the group project, teams of students analyzed a specific family policy issue and developed a "change strategy" for dealing with a specific family or child policy issue at the agency or community level. The curriculum prepared students for these projects by going into detail on the policymaking process. Readings highlighted policymaking techniques and skills such as persuasion, coalition building, letter-writing campaigns, and testifying before committees.

Endersby and Webber (1995) report on a semester-long project in which undergraduates took on roles of policymakers, lobbyists, and members of Congress. They researched and prepared briefs, memos, and bills using email and message boards to communicate progress to students with different roles in other classes. The simulation culminated in a two-day long mock Congress.

The goals of active learning also emphasize critical thinking. Definitions of critical thinking vary, but most characterize it as "the intentional application of rational, higher order thinking skills, such as analysis, synthesis, problem recognition and problem solving, inference, and evaluation" (Angelo, 1995, p. 6). Critical thinking is viewed as one of the basic competencies every college graduate should have (Diamond, 1997). Asay and Curry (2003) outline a critical thinking project for marriage and family students in which they solve problems related to a family-centered personal or societal problem. The steps of the project reflect the necessary skills for policy making, which is really problem-solving on a societal scale. The steps include: identifying a problem; gathering information and research on the topic; generating a "perfect world" solution; formulating several possible realistic solutions; choosing one workable solution; constructing an action plan; and reflecting on the problem solving process.

Other elements of family policy curricula devoted to active, contextual learning include: internships (Cohen et al., 1995), observing local government sessions, letter writing to public officials, working directly with community advocacy agencies, discussing family policy in current events (Anderson & Skinner, 1995), cooperative learning exercises and class discussion of case law (Henderson & Martin, 2002).

## *Motivation*

Successful instructors often attempt to get students excited about the material by "sharing" their field and experiences with them, so that they in turn will explore areas that are valuable for their own career, educational development, and the betterment of the community (Scheckley & Keeton, 1997). When students are asked questions and encounter complexity, they become more curious and intrinsically motivated (McKeachie, 1994). Students must be given challenging tasks, with reasonable risks. In order to give them a chance to succeed, they must also be provided with structure (e.g., examples; incremental due dates) and feedback to help them improve their performance (McKeachie, 1994; Tuckman, 2003).

## *Writing Skills for the Policy Arena*

Anderson and Skinner (1995) note that a person beginning a career in social policy must have exceptional writing skills. "Policy writing is often different from the style learned by most students in writing term papers. Policy writing reflects a style more closely aligned with the principles offered in journalism. . . . Likewise, being able to transmit information orally in a succinct and interesting style is a skill that needs to be developed" (p. 73).

This type of policy (and legal) brief writing is a core feature in the course described in this paper. Students were taught that briefs that summarize and critique existing research can help to inform policy or law at any stage, from identifying a problem to an extensive evaluation of existing policy. Policy briefs may be used to influence policymaking of legislative or funding bodies. Similarly, an *amicus curiae* (friend of the court) brief summarizing research and recommending a course of action to the courts may take the form of an objective "science translation" brief or an "advocacy brief" (Monroe, 1995; Roesch, Golding, Hans, & Reppucci, 1991). Social scientists have much to offer to policy/law, provided that they are clear about their biases and role conflicts and can offer an objective conclusion about the state-of-the-art in their field of research (Bazelon, 1982). It can, of course, be difficult work. "To be useful, family scientists must strike a balance between presenting disputed research as fact versus presenting a paralyzing statement of indecision" (Monroe, 1991, p. 328).

In terms of objectivity, science translation briefs have several possible advantages over expert testimony. Brief writers, in contrast to many expert witnesses, are not paid for their work. Science translation briefs document sources and present conclusions formed by a critique of the available research base (i.e., strengths and weaknesses of theory, method, and interpretation). When a brief is submitted by a scientific organization (e.g., the American Psychology-Law Society), a broad range of research is reviewed and "the courts may have more confidence that the brief represents the field as a whole" (Roesch et al., 1991, p. 4). In summary, brief writing is an important skill for social scientists whose work has implications for law and policy.

## Evaluation of Policy/Law Courses

Consistent with many recent calls for instructional evaluation (e.g., Murray, 1999), we feel that assessment and feedback are important for ongoing course development. Why is assessment of curricular and instructional impact important? The answer is simple: educational accountability and professional credibility. We can regularly evaluate whether our curriculum and educational interventions make a difference to the student learner/consumer.

Most educational authorities agree that assessing curricular and instructional impact is one critical way to bring respect and credibility to academic units and institutions in higher education (Murray, 1999). There is a clear need to design courses and curricula to reflect core competencies and to evaluate instructional impact to determine whether students are meeting the objectives set for students (Diamond, 1997; Murray, 1999).

At the individual course level, some policy instructors have collected evaluation data from their students. Keller et al. (2001), for example, discuss the reactions of 44 second-year MSW students involved in a debating curriculum. Analysis showed that students' topical knowledge increased significantly from pre- to post-test. Students reported a greater increase in knowledge associated with debate topics than they reported for topics covered via traditional instruction. In addition, students reported a greater increase in knowledge for the topic they debated as opposed to topics covered by other classmates' debates.

Rocha and Johnson (1997) also elicited reactions from social work students in a policy course. Although their data collection process feedback was more informal than Keller et al.'s (2001) evaluation, the students' comments reflect an achievement of many of the course goals described in the literature review above. These comments, which reflect student feedback from 1992 to 1997, include: experiential work as enhancing the level of learning; student empowerment; increased public speaking confidence; exposure to a variety of problem solving tactics; and the acquisition of policy practice knowledge and skills.

Markus, Howard, and King (1993) examined the educational value of service learning by incorporating service learning into a large undergraduate political science course. Two of eight discussion sections were assigned as "community service" sections. These students were required to do 20 hours of service and the students' experiences were discussed in section meetings. The other six sections were devoted to traditional discussions of readings and lectures. Students in the service learning sections had significantly higher grades and reported more often that, through the course, they had developed the ability to apply principles they learned, they had a greater awareness of societal problems, and they acquired a greater sense of personal responsibility.

Anderson and Skinner (1995) suggest that family policy courses follow one of two formats–either "topical" (i.e., focusing on actual policies relating to various family and social issues) or "process" (i.e., focusing on the process by which policies are created and enforced). The course we describe in this paper attempts to do both, in an effort to stimulate interest in law and policy among human development and family studies students.

## COURSE DESCRIPTION

### Course Objectives

We now describe a course taught in the School of Family Studies at the University of Connecticut. As stated on the syllabus for the undergraduate and graduate versions of "Child Welfare, Law, and Social Policy," the goals of the class are to acquaint students with:

- Various areas in which public policies and laws affect children and families, and in which family/social science research and practice are germane to legal policy (and case law);
- The methods through which empirical research findings may influence case law and legislation (*amicus curiae* and policy briefs);
- Intensive, empirical examinations of contemporary social problems that relate to children and families;
- The relationship between the fields of family studies/social science, policy, and law, and how this knowledge can affect study design and dissemination.

Key areas of focus include: primary prevention vs. secondary and tertiary intervention approaches to promoting child/family welfare and mental health; policies and services directed toward individuals with special needs; and, family violence prevention and intervention efforts.

Examples of case law and pieces of legislation are used to explain the development and application of laws, as well as the ways in which changing societal values are reflected in the legal realm. For example, one case that we discuss is *DeShaney v. Winnebago County Social Services Department* (1989). This case deals with a 4-year-old child beaten repeatedly and severely by his father. Although the Department had documented numerous instances of suspected abuse, the child was never removed. When the child's (non-custodial) mother finally brought suit against the Department for negligence, the court ruled that the Department was not responsible for the child's injury, because he had never been in the state's custody. This case shows students how, at times, our societal values (e.g., against child abuse) are at odds with the technicalities of written law. It also provides opportunities to debate and write on the interrelated interests of child, parent, and state, custody arrangements, and appropriate child welfare practices. For example, a brief could be used to argue for a clearer focus on the interests of children in such cases (see Crosby-Currie & Reppucci, 1999).

The Adoption and Safe Families Act (ASFA) of 1997 is discussed as a piece of legislation that conflicts, in part, with the realities of families in crisis. We might argue that ASFA's emphasis on permanence through adoption is antithetical to the temporary nature of foster care, creating an environment that minimizes biological parents' opportunities to be rehabilitated and reunited with their children.

Promoting adoption supports the research that says children suffer from "foster care drift" (i.e., the physical and psychological instability characteristic of long-term involvement in state custody and/or multiple transitions), but it ignores family-preservation research emphasizing biological parents' potential to maintain safe homes. In this way, ASFA highlights the ways in which laws are built on empirical research, yet it also points out the ways in which laws may serve some family research interests over others.

## Graded Assignments

With an emphasis on skill building, final grades in the undergraduate course are determined by students' performance on a mid-term exam, final exam, class participation, written legal and policy briefs, and the oral presentation of a brief. Students were given grading criteria for all assignments in advance. See Tables 1 and 2 for grading criteria for the written brief assignments (policy and *amicus curiae* briefs) and the oral presentation of the briefs, respectively. All of the graded elements for each assignment are viewed as important; as such, they are weighted equally. Detailed written feedback on each of the assignments is also important to the students' learning and motivation.

*Research paper.* In lieu of the two exams, the graduate course has a requirement of a 15-page literature review paper (due early in the semester), which serves as a basis for the briefs. This paper is a *critical review* of the scientific psychological literature on the topic of the student's choice. The suggested structure for the paper includes: a critical review of the available literature (noting strengths and limitations of research methodology); conclusions about what is known from the convergent findings, and what is still not conclusively known; and, recommendations for future research. Students with limited experience in writing literature review articles are directed to several sources, including Bem (1995), for guidelines.

*Amicus curiae brief.* Having become "expert" on a psychological/family studies topic relevant to the law by virtue of writing the review paper (for graduate students) or researching, outlining, and discussing a

TABLE 1. Written Legal or Policy Brief Grading Criteria

Quality of Content
- _____ Logical argument is made, cohesively
- _____ Good use of relevant research articles (esp. primary, empirical articles)–but with a focus on just a few key articles for purposes of the brief
- _____ Well integrated: demonstrates good understanding of the topic; research is critiqued and cited articles are integrated, rather than summarized
- _____ Statements supported with references to a few key research studies, etc.
- _____ References are strong (journal articles? government statistics?), relevant

Organization
- _____ Clear statement of the issue
- _____ Critical review of the literature (noting strengths and limitations of research methodology)
- _____ Conclusions about what is known (and not yet known) from convergent findings
- _____ Clear recommendations for action relevant to the court case, policy, etc.

Quality of Writing
- _____ Written for the lay person (or appropriate judge[s], policymakers), assuming no previous knowledge of family studies research
- _____ Follows APA (5th ed.) style, with in-text citations and references at the end
- _____ Objective and scientific: doesn't go beyond the data in statements or conclusions
- _____ Nicely written: spelling, punctuation, sentence structure, style

topic with classmates and the instructor (for undergraduates), students are then charged to translate their findings into a recommendation for a judge who is hearing a case. In just 5-7 double-spaced pages, students are asked to present: an introduction to the issue (e.g., should a 5-yr-old's testimony be admissible?), and how it is directly relevant to the case at hand; a short summary of the research findings (including "both sides" as applicable); a conclusion about what the research suggests (and limitations); and, a direct recommendation to a judge about what s/he should do in this case. The brief should be written for the lay person, assuming no previous knowledge of family studies research. However, statements should be backed up with references to a few key research studies. This assignment represents the kind of brief that might be submitted by a guardian *ad litem* on behalf of a child, or by a professional as "expert" testimony.

*Policy brief.* A policy briefing memo is one of the major forms of communication between legislators and their staff; it is also used for translating research for a variety of applied audiences. The construction

TABLE 2. Oral Presentation Grading Criteria

Organization
- _____ Logically organized?
- _____ Addressed the class as a specific, appropriate policy audience
- _____ Ends with clear recommendation?

Quality of Content
- _____ Research base is convincing, strong, and valid
- _____ Logical application of research to argument
- _____ Sound conclusions (recommendations)

Preparation
- _____ 5 minutes = 5 minutes
- _____ Handouts ___ overheads ___ slides ___ probing questions ___ other

Presentation/Facilitation Skills
- _____ Appropriate use of technology, *if* technology is used
- _____ Speaker is professional
- _____ Appropriate tone (no jargon, but sufficiently formal)
- _____ Effective presentation skills (appears practiced/polished)
- _____ Fielded questions effectively during 3 minutes of questions

of such a document, after an extensive review of the research literature, provides the student with practice in preparing a succinct summary of information for practitioners and policy makers. The memo should address a specific issue on which an intervention or policy is being considered. Similar to the court brief, the task is to: summarize the issue; present the relevant perspectives and the associated research support; and, make a recommendation for action. One key is to remember the audience.

For example, in a policy brief relating to ASFA, one student proposed changes to the U.S. Department of Health & Human Services, Administration for Children & Families that would increase federal financial support for reunification efforts for biological parents.

*Oral presentation.* At the end of the semester, students have 5 minutes in class to present one of their briefs orally, as if the class was the legislative body, community entity, or judge(s) that they seek to address. The students then field questions from the class for 3 minutes.

## Teaching Evaluations as an Outcome

Students' end-of-the-semester teaching evaluations are often used to assess their satisfaction with the course and instructor. There is much debate as to the validity of these ratings for tapping "effective" teaching (e.g., McKeachie, 1994), but they do provide one barometer of "success."

*Quantitative feedback.* Students rate instructors/courses on 11 dimensions in courses (undergraduate and graduate) at the University of Connecticut. The rated dimensions are: presented material effectively; organization; clear objectives; fulfilled objectives; clear assignments; stimulated interest; graded fairly; appropriate exam; accessibility; shows interest, concern; preparation. Ratings range from 1 ("Unacceptable") to 10 ("Outstanding").

The mean for these 11 ratings for the course is 9.7. This rating is fairly consistent over five undergraduate (range of 8 to 45 students; mean = 25) and three graduate (range of 6-10 students; mean = 8) course offerings from 1998 to 2003. At face value, the high scores suggest that students were satisfied with the course's organization, assignments, and objectives.

*Qualitative feedback.* Over the years, a number of undergraduates have stated that although the class required the most work or writing or–gasp!–thinking of any course they have taken, they have learned the most, liked the class the most, and/or found the class to be most relevant to their future work as any class they have taken.

Students in the Fall 2003 graduate course and Winter 2003 undergraduate course were asked to provide written feedback on their experiences of the course, including the writing and presentation of their briefs, at the completion of the class. There were several recurring themes in the students' responses. We present those themes, and some exemplary quotes, in terms of perceived challenges, issues related to the process of translating research, and outcomes.

*Challenges.* Students, especially the undergraduates, appreciated being able to choose their own topics. They reported that it made the work more enjoyable and motivated them to dig deeper into the issue. At the same time, many students were anxious about trying a new form of writing, about presenting in front of the class, and about having to "take a stand" rather than simply summarize research. Students were uncertain of their skills at the beginning of these assignments.

> One aspect of the process that I found to be difficult was viewing myself as someone who is knowledgeable enough about a topic to write briefs and recommendations. [Graduate Student]

> Once I read the syllabus and saw that we had to do some sort of writing that I had no experience with, I got scared. Then as I read on and saw that we had an oral presentation, too, I thought I was doomed for failure. [Undergraduate Student]

> I think [the oral presentation] was the best of all the assignments of the semester. It forced us to be concise and diplomatic while also demonstrating our passion for the topic. [Graduate Student]

*Translating research.* For many students, the concept of a research paper was familiar. Translation from research to brief, however, was challenging. Students found it difficult to be concise and write without employing research jargon.

> In some respects, the legal brief/oral presentation assignment was similar to other assignments I have had, and in other respects, it was very different. . ... Both involved evaluating the research on a specific topic and then integrating the various materials. The similarity made the research aspect of the assignment and some of the writing aspect easier. [Undergraduate Student]

> It was difficult to whittle my original literature review to the bare essentials and translate the findings from jargon to more accessible language. [Graduate Student]

> I thought it was extremely beneficial to have the research paper on the topic already completed. Writing the research paper early in the semester . . . provided me with ample time to really analyze the literature on the topic and get a good feel for what the literature reveals and how it should best be applied. [Graduate Student]

> Translating this brief from the research paper was challenging in terms of trying to maintain a very clear focus on my goal of receiving funding for a particular research study. [Graduate Student]

The students also showed a bit of savvy in understanding the importance of adding a compelling story, a sobering statistic, or a real face to go with their data-based review of research findings on their chosen topic.

> I added a story about a real girl that went through the struggles of medical treatment and informed consent. I wanted to get the audience to care about the girl and use it to see the idea of informed consent from my point of view. [Undergraduate Student]

*Limitations in depth.* Rocha and Johnson (1997) note that there are limitations to what can be covered in a given course and that choices must be made between broader versus deeper coverage of family policy topics. That is certainly true for the course we describe.

> The wide range of subjects gave my classmates and me an excellent overview of policy issues affecting children. The downside to this breadth of information, of course, is that we were limited in our investigation of each of these topics; each of the topics we covered could easily be taught as an entire course. [Graduate Student]

*Outcomes.* By the end of the course, every student reported learning a great deal from the brief-writing exercises. Many reported that, in spite of their initial fear of the unknown, they emerged from the course with a feeling of "empowerment" or an increase in confidence.

> ... it was a great feeling to realize that ... I did know a great deal about the topic and my opinion and recommendations would be research informed and empirically based. [Graduate Student]

> This assignment was unique in that it taught me that anyone, if they have the passion, motivation, and the means to present a case could make a difference in the world. People can change juries' opinions or strengthen weak cases. Prior to this assignment, I always believed that older adults that have established themselves in a profession or are famous for whatever reason were the only people that could change laws or regulations or propose new ones. Now I see that if someone wants to implement change you have to have a good case, have research to support your case and be able to present it in a clear fashion. [Undergraduate Student]

Students reported that the course increased their knowledge of their topics, and helped them develop research, brief writing, and presentation skills. Students ended the course feeling confident in their ability to participate in the policymaking process.

> I feel after completion of the course that I now possess the skills to thoroughly research, evaluate and extract the most important aspects of a topic. This, along with the knowledge and experience of formatting and presenting briefs leaves me feeling well equipped to write an effective brief on a topic of interest. [Graduate Student]

> ... I think that after experiencing firsthand the research, writing, and translation process of a particular topic that I am more knowledgeable about policy briefs and the process that is necessary for their construction. [Graduate Student]

Several students commented that brief writing and presenting were helpful and exciting methods of learning. They appreciated the practical application of information, and they gained a sense of how research studies are put to use in the real world.

> Writing the *amicus curiae* brief and the policy brief as well as putting together the presentation for the class ... forced me to get inside the research in a unique and relevant way. [Graduate Student]

> I think it is very progressive for a family studies program to teach its students how to collaborate with different kinds of professionals. This class helped me to broaden my definition of a social scientist's purpose ... [Graduate Student]

## CONCLUSION

We present a promising approach to teaching marriage and family students about policy/law relevant issues. The idea of brief writing and oral presentations in a family policy course is hardly new (e.g., Rocha & Johnson, 1997), but the literature on its effectiveness is limited. We report findings from the open-ended responses of undergraduate and graduate students to an active learning course on Child Welfare, Law, and Social Policy.

Further research on the effectiveness of this kind of course will require more formal evaluation. Outcomes such as civic engagement and competence in writing or orally presenting research findings, in addition to standardized assessments of critical thinking ability, may be of interest. This work fits, in the long run, within a larger framework of assessing impact on students' experiences–building a demographic, experiential, educational profile of students as they enter, encounter, and exit our program. Who are our students? What do we do with them? How do they experience it? What do they learn? What do they do next? In other words, do we make a difference?

Our simple, qualitative data do not allow us to address whether the course has made such an impact. We also do not have feedback from time points throughout the semester in order to address the impact of specific assignments. At this point, however, we can feel comfortable suggesting that student ratings and open-ended comments on an assessment of end-of-the-semester reactions to the assignments support the notion that the course and assignments challenged the students. They also emerged from the course reporting that they had developed skills, confidence, and an appreciation for the interplay between law, policy, and the social sciences.

On a broader level, the course described here represents a model for promoting students' critical thinking and engagement in science translation or advocacy. The written and oral simulations conducted in the course offer both undergraduate and graduate participants the opportunity to engage in problem solving with some real-world constraints. Though the assignments allow for some degree of creativity, students are compelled to present policy recommendations in a way digestible for *other* consumers (i.e., judges, legislators, bureaucrats, practitioners). Students must communicate their platform yet rein in their passion or opinions in order to be persuasive within the parameters of our social policymaking system. In this way, the brief writing and oral presentations help develop students' scientific research *and* lay communication skills. Such skills are critical not only for students who may pursue careers in marriage and family policy and law, but also for any student who hopes to cultivate change in our society.

## REFERENCES

Adoption and Safe Families Act (1997), *P.L. 105-89.*
Anderson, E. A., & Skinner, D. A. (1995). The components of family policy education. *Journal of Family and Economic Issues, 16*, 65-77.
Angelo, T. A. (1995). Classroom assessment for critical thinking. *Teaching of Psychology, 22*, 6-7.

Asay, S. M., & Curry, B. M. (2003). Implementing and assessing a critical thinking problem solving project. *Journal of Teaching in Marriage & Family, 3,* 375-398.

Bazelon, D. L. (1982). Veils, values, and social responsibility. *American Psychologist, 37,* 115-121.

Bem, D. J. (1995). Writing a review article for Psychological Bulletin. *Psychological Bulletin, 118,* 172-177.

Bogenschneider, K. (2002). *Family policy matters: How policymaking affects families and what professionals can do.* Mahwah, NJ: Erlbaum.

Boyd, S. B. (1989). Teaching policy issues in family law. *Canadian Journal of Family Law, 8,* 11-15.

Brunner, R. D. (1997). Teaching the policy sciences: Reflections on a graduate seminar. *Policy Sciences, 30,* 217-231.

Cohen, S., Eimicke, W., & Ukeles, J. (1995). Teaching the craft of policy and management analysis: The workshop sequence at Columbia University's graduate program in public policy and administration. *Journal of Policy Analysis and Management, 14,* 606-626.

Crosby-Currie, C., & Reppucci, N. D. (1999). The missing child in child protection: The Constitutional context of child maltreatment from *Meyer* to *DeShaney. Law & Policy, 21,* 129-159.

*DeShaney v. Winnebago County Social Services Department* (1989). 489, U.S. 189.

Diamond, R.M. (1997). Broad curriculum reform is needed if students are to master core skills. T*he Chronicle of Higher Education, August 1,* B7.

Endersby, J. W., & Webber, D. J. (1995). Iron triangle simulation: A role-playing game for undergraduates in Congress, interest groups, and public policy classes. *Political Science & Politics, 28,* 520-523.

Henderson, T. L., & Martin, K. J. (2002). Cooperative learning as one approach to teaching family law. *Family Relations, 51,* 351-360.

Huber, M. T. (2004). *Balancing acts: The scholarship of teaching and learning in academic careers.* Washington, DC: American Association for Higher Education and The Carnegie Foundation for the Advancement of Teaching.

Keller, T. E., Whittaker, J. K., & Burke, T. K. (2001). Student debates in policy courses: Promoting policy practice skills and knowledge through active learning. *Journal of Social Work Education, 37,* 343-355.

Markus, G. B., Howard, J. P. F., & King, D. C. (1993). Integrating community service and classroom instruction enhances learning: Results from an experiment. *Educational Evaluation and Policy Analysis, 15,* 410-419.

McKeachie, W. J. (1994). *Teaching tips: Strategies, research, and theory for college and university teachers (9th* ed.). Lexington, MA: D. C. Heath & Company.

Melton, G. B. (Ed.) (1987). *Reforming the law: Impact of child development research.* New York: Guilford Publications.

Monroe, P. A. (1991). Participation in state legislative activities: A practical guide for family scientists. *Family Relations, 40,* 324-331.

Monroe, P. A. (1995). Family policy advocacy: Putting knowledge to work. *Family Relations, 44,* 425-437.

Murray, B. (1999). Rising costs press faculty to account for students' learning. *American Psychological Association Monitor, April,* 33-34.

Reppucci, N. D., & Aber, M. (1987). Views of public policy psychologists. *The Clinical Psychologist, Spring*, 36-38.

Rickel, A. U., & Becker, E. (1997). *Keeping children from harm's way: How national policy affects psychological development.* Washington, DC: American Psychological Association.

Rocha, C. J., & Johnson, A. K. (1997). Teaching family policy through a policy practice framework. *Journal of Social Work Education, 33*, 433-444.

Roesch, R., Golding, S. L., Hans, V. P., & Reppucci, N. D. (1991). Social science and the courts: The role of *amicus curiae* briefs. *Law and Human Behavior, 15*, 1-11.

Scheckley, B. G., & Keeton, M. T. (1997). Service learning: A theoretical model. In J. Schine (Ed.), *Service Learning: Ninety-sixth yearbook of the National Society for the Study of Education, Part 1* (pp. 32-55). Chicago, IL: University of Chicago Press.

Tuckman, B. W. (2003). The effect of learning and motivation strategies on college students' achievement. *Journal of College Student Development, 4*, 430-437.

# Family Law and Foster Care: Cooperative Research Teams

Tammy L. Henderson
Lenore McWey

**ABSTRACT.** There are challenges associated with teaching family law and public policy; however, cooperative learning, a recognized teaching strategy that serves to enhance students' overall development, including academic, cognitive, and social growth, can be used successfully to teach this subject matter. In this paper, we describe how we taught students about some aspects of qualitative research methods, foster care policies, and pertinent family law concepts and practices; this was done through the initiation of a research team of undergraduate and graduate students. We explain the development of a cooperative research team, and the methods used to teach family law, using foster care as a context. The observed outcomes for students and faculty members are offered to readers. *[Article copies available for a fee from The Haworth Document Delivery Service: 1-800-HAWORTH. E-mail address: <docdelivery@haworthpress.com> Website: <http://www.HaworthPress.com> © 2005 by The Haworth Press, Inc. All rights reserved.]*

**KEYWORDS.** Cooperative learning, cooperative research teams, family law, foster care, research teams.

---

Tammy L. Henderson is Assistant Professor, Department of Human Development, Virginia Polytechnic Institute and State University (Virginia Tech). Lenore McWey is Assistant Professor, Florida State University.

Address correspondence to: Tammy L. Henderson, Human Development (0416), Blacksburg, VA 24061 (E-mail: thender@vt.edu).

© 2005 by The Haworth Press, Inc. All rights reserved.
doi:10.1300/J002v38n02_03

## INTRODUCTION

The challenges associated with teaching family law in family science, human development, and related programs are multifaceted. First, family law typically is associated with explicit issues of marriage, sexual relationships (i.e., incest, sodomy laws, and the like), parenthood (i.e., adoption and parental rights), family disruption (i.e., divorce, child support, alimony, and pre- and postnuptial agreements), and child maltreatment. Yet, family law also involves implicit policies that shape behaviors and relationships within and outside of the family, including but not limited to traffic laws, zoning ordinances (i.e., *Moore v. the City of East Cleveland*, 1977), and more. Because family law involves both implicit and explicit domains, capturing the complexities and intersections of family development and family law can be a test for family researchers, practitioners, and educators.

A second challenge is that few family scientists are trained to teach or conduct research related to family law or have had courses in this subject area. Most family science and related programs offer only one course on family policy or law, or some combination of family law and policy. Furthermore, there may be few opportunities for faculty to learn about changes within various policy arenas, such as state and federal legislation, judicial decisions, and administrative regulations and policies. Family law, may be less familiar to professionals in human development, family studies, and related disciplines (Anderson & Skinner, 1995); yet, it remains an important domain for scholarly and instructional exploration.

Third, we believe that teaching family law supports efforts to build a larger group of learned, involved citizens, helps students to move research to practice, and cultivates the scholarship of social science professionals in the area of family law. In fact, developing a cadre of upcoming scholars and practitioners who understand the influence of laws on family development and vice versa (Tanke & Tanke, 1979; Walters, 1983) requires innovative and deliberate instructional approaches. We suggest looking beyond traditional pedagogies (i.e., lecture) and using research teams based on cooperative learning strategies as a way to teach family law. Below we briefly explain the pedagogy of cooperative learning, review the details of our cooperative learning research team, and highlight the outcomes for students and faculty.

## DEFINING COOPERATIVE LEARNING

Traditional approaches to teaching family policy or law involve students attending class, listening to lectures, reading textbooks and articles, and sometimes making legislative or courtroom visits. However, it has been stated that teaching policy in the traditional format is challenging because students often do not see the immediate relevance of the impact of policies or laws and often feel removed from the content (Cianciolo & Henderson, 2003). Thus, teaching family law, like family policy, requires innovative teaching strategies (Cianciolo & Henderson, 2003; Cianciolo, Henderson, Kretzer, & Mendes, 2001) like cooperative learning (CL). CL is the use of small groups of students working together to take full advantage of their own and each other's knowledge (Dunlap & Grabinger, 1996; Johnson, Johnson, & Smith, 1991).

It has been stated that CL strategies are superior to traditional classroom approaches because they have been shown to enhance students academic, social, and cognitive outcomes, including team-building skills (Cohen & Lotan, 1997; Cianciolo et al., 2001; Lotan & Whitcomb, 1998; Nokinske & Millis, 1997; Slavin, 1995a, 1995b; Sharin, 1994; Stevens & Slavin, 1995; Walker, 1996), with effective planning by instructors (Steiner, Stromwall, Brzuzy, & Gerdes, 1999). Other advantages of CL are well documented. For example, this pedagogical approach enhances student achievement and interpersonal relationships among group members, as well as improves the retention rates of students (Kluge, 1990; Totten, Sills, & Digby, 1991). CL provides students with increased opportunities for discussion, shared learning, and self-management based on their academic strengths (Slavin & Cooper, 1999). This pedagogical strategy also complements an interdisciplinary approach to teaching and learning, exposing students to family science, marriage and family therapy, family law, policy sciences, and other disciplines. As such, an interdisciplinary approach is more likely to have familiar content, appealing to a broader range of students (Dinmore, 1997) whose personal or academic experiences may differ.

Four types of cooperative learning groups are available when designing a research team: (a) *completely cooperative groups* operate to jointly reach group goals and complete cooperative group assignments (Stodolsky, 1984); (b) *cooperative groups* have collective goals and course assignments with individually assigned tasks; (c) *helping obligatory CL groups* have individual goals and assignments; (d) the *helping permitted groups* have individual goals and course assignments with limited student interactions, strictly determined by the student.

## THE COOPERATIVE RESEARCH TEAM

Serving as monitors and coaches, we used *cooperative groups,* to educate students about research related to families directly involved in the foster care system. Specifically, the focus of the research project was to explore the legal reasoning used to terminate the rights of parents whose children were in the foster care system. We also hoped that cooperative groups, referred to in this paper as cooperative research teams, would better prepare undergraduate students for graduate studies, assist graduate students in enhancing their other research endeavors, expand students' applied skills, and support them in identifying potential career paths focused on family law or policy.

Generally, our cooperative research team was shaped by (a) shared goals and rewards, (b) the tasks of coding and verifying data using Grounded Theory Methods, (c) learning how to effectively use Word, Excel, and Power Point, and (d) participating in research team meetings to discuss new themes, coding challenges, and family law precedents in foster care cases (e.g., Goodwin, 1999; Johnson, Johnson, Holubec, & Roy, 1994; Nolinske & Mills, 1997). Our cooperative learning research team capitalized on diversity, heterogeneous learning styles, and the individual strengths of each member, making it possible for students to learn the value of teamwork, and to collaborate and negotiate professional and personal success while working with individuals from diverse backgrounds (Nolinske & Mills, 1997). Like any cooperative group, shared responsibility rather than individual competition (Goodwin, 1999; Nolinske & Mills, 1997) was emphasized. Faculty members monitored students' progress and worked with them to establish professional expectations, to reduce the incidence of workhorses and dominators, and to lessen the incidence of any unhealthy competitive behaviors that undermine the success of the team.

Our cooperative research team was comprised of six undergraduate students, two graduate students, and two faculty members. All of the undergraduate students were juniors or seniors majoring in Human Development, with an interest in attending graduate school. The graduate students were pursuing doctoral degrees. Both graduate students were in the same department but had different majors; one was studying Family Studies and the other Marriage and Family Therapy. Finally, two faculty colleagues who were in the same department directed the team for most of the experience; however, one member relocated at the end of the first academic year. One faculty member's expertise lies in the area of Marriage and Family Therapy and foster care research. The other faculty member teaches in the Family Studies area and specializes in family policy and law research.

## PREPARING FOR THE COOPERATIVE RESEARCH EXPERIENCE

Planning and implementing a 15-week research experience is critical for effective CL environments, although most students may enroll in research courses for more than one semester. Planning began with an assessment of the goals for the project. One primary focus of the research team was to teach students how to conduct research; the primary student objective was to enhance their research competencies. Other student objectives included expectations that undergraduate and graduate students would learn: (a) how judicial decision-making shapes family development and how families shape judicial decision-making; (b) how courts regulate, orchestrate, support, or hinder family wellness for foster care families; and (c) how to master skills, such as critical thinking and evaluation skills for today's technological, service, and information-based economy.

To accomplish the student objectives, we had to ensure that students could deconstruct, reconstruct, and review the legal and familial issues that emerged in the data, which were foster care court cases. For example, in order for students to understand how parents with mental health challenges lost their parental rights, we examined court decisions and acknowledged the significance of justices' interpretation of the Adoption and Safe Family Act (ASFA, PL 105-89) of 1997 and related laws. The Adoption and Safe Family Act (ASFA) has a requirement that parents demonstrate improvement in the factors that lead to the removal of their children from the home within a period of 12 to 18 months after the intervention by social services. Recognizing, for example, that mentally challenged parents might not be able to show substantial improvements in their intellectual and emotional capacities within the legally defined period, the research team was able to see the incongruence between decisions based on developmental trajectories versus those made strictly by legal precedents or the strict reading of the law.

The authors extracted cases from LEXIS NEXIS, an electronic database of legal articles and court opinions, to secure foster care cases in the state of Virginia. After accessing state case law for Virginia, we extracted cases that were decided between January 1, 1960 and December 10, 2002. The initial date corresponded with child welfare policies that focused on the Battered-Child Syndrome, the war on poverty, and part of the Civil Rights era in the United States, whereas the ending date marked the cessation of the data collection process. Consequently, we found a population of state supreme court ($N = 15$) and appellate court cases ($N = 168$). The rationale for the sampling procedure, referred to as theoretical sampling (Creswell, 1998; Strauss & Corbin, 1990), was explained to the research team during the orientation; these details were placed in a handout given to team members.

In preparation for the transition into a complex, multi-site research project with one primary researcher relocating at the end of the academic year, we attended to some administrative tasks necessary to manage the data, and an ongoing research project. Using Microsoft Word, we listed the cases being used in the study. We gave each case an identification number, recorded the history and facts of the case, identified the gender of the parent whose parental rights were at risk of being terminated, cataloged the decision regarding parental rights, explained the legal issues presented in the case, and established the ruling or decision (see Table 1). To verify students coding of the data, we used an Excel file to list the identification number for each case, recording other pertinent information (for example, primary parental issue manifested in the case, gender of the parent appealing the decision to terminate parental rights [TPR], court ruling, and whether the court ruling occurred before or after the enactment of Adoption and Safe Family Act; see Table 2). Additional clarification of Tables 1 and 2 are given later in this paper.

## *Orientation*

Prior to beginning the research process, the research team met for an orientation. We discussed student objectives, research goals, general expectations, and assessment processes used to evaluate students' learning. Because students enrolled for one to three credit hours, we had to clearly define the basis of assessment. Students understood that they were being assessed on their research team meeting attendance, quality of work, and their ability to effectively collaborate and support the efforts of the team. We discussed end of term requirements, such as the final narrative and other items discussed in the outcomes section of this paper.

During orientation, we provided each cooperative research team member with a packet of information. The packets included articles, relevant handouts, instructions on creating tables and data files, coding guidelines, and legal terms and precedents. Packets also included an ar-

TABLE 1. Excerpt from Thematic Coding Structure Used by CL Research Team

| ID No. | Descriptive Codes |
|---|---|
| ID No. | Case Number |
| Facts | Why Child Placed in Foster Care? |
| | Background/History of Case–facts of the case |
| | Gender of Parent–the parent or parents before the court |
| | Family Risk and Protective Factors of Parents (ex: poverty, mental or physical disabilities, work skills, education, and other factors) |
| | Physical Health or Disabilities of Parent; Physical Health or Disabilities of the Child |
| | Mental Illness of Parent–PROBES: depression, self injuring behavior |
| | Mental Illness of Child |
| | Risk and Protective Factors for the Child–PROBES: child abuse, neglect, sexual abuse, or developmental challenges |
| Legal Issues | Best Interests of the Child–threat of harm to the child, unfit parents, or other developmental reasons |
| | Parental Rights and Family Autonomy |
| | Standard of Review–Clear and Convincing Evidence |
| | Procedure Due Process–right to be heard, represented, and notification or adherence to the foster care, child abuse, and other laws, such as compliance with foster care plan |
| | Termination of Parental Rights |
| Legal Terms | Parens patriae, ore tenuous, privacy rights, liberty interests, fundamental right, etc. |
| Ruling | Decision by Court |
| Coder | Name of student |
| Verifier | Name of student |

ticle in which scholars used Grounded Theory Methods (Creswell, 1998; Strauss & Corbin, 1990) to study holiday letters (Banks, Louie, & Einerson, 2000), providing an overview of this form of qualitative data analysis. We discussed the packet contents and provided directives for analyzing data using Grounded Theory Method (GTM) and mastering word processing, spreadsheet software, and Power Point. For example, during orientation we provided an introduction to family law and foster care laws, including a review of the handout of legal terms and precedents. This review of legal terms and precedents proved to be extremely important because it not only introduced critical legal tests and terms, but also helped students understand the constraints of the judicial system and the intersecting relationship of family development and law.

TABLE 2. Example of Excel Sheet Data–Primary Coding System

| ID | Parental Issue | Gender | Decision | Pre-ASFA | Post-ASFA |
|---|---|---|---|---|---|
| 11 | Jail | Female | TPR | | X |
| 12 | Non-Compliance | Female | TPR | | X |
| 13 | Neglect | Male | TPR | | X |
| 14 | Mentally Challenged | Female | Reversed | X | |
| 15 | Jail | Female | TPR | | X |
| 16 | Mental Health | Male/Female | TPR | X | |
| 17 | Substance Abuse | Female | TPR | | X |
| 18 | Substance Abuse/Neglect | Male | TPR | | X |
| 19 | Mental Health/Neglect | Female | TPR | X | |
| 20 | Substance Abuse/Jail | Female | TPR | | X |
| 21 | Neglect | Female | TPR | | X |
| 22 | Non-TPR Case | N/A | N/A | X | |
| 23 | Substance Abuse/Neglect | Female | TPR | | X |
| 24 | Non-Compliance | Female | TPR | | X |

Above is an excerpt of the Excel sheet used to categorize data. TPR = Termination of parental rights. Pre-ASFA refers to those cases decided before the implementation of the Adoption and Safe Families Act. Post-ASFA refers to cases decided after the implementation of the Adoption and Safe Families Act.

Students were able to review how justices interpret legislative acts, and to identify the thinking of the courts in contrast to that of family scientists, practitioners, and educators. The review of legal terms and court cases were critical aspects of the work of the research team.

Given the page constraints for publications, we present excerpts of this coding schema in Table 1. Students were given the coding schema to interpret and code the data found in court cases related to foster care. They were asked to read the case several times and determine the following: (a) why the child was placed in foster care, (b) what were the facts of the case, (c) did the child or parents have any specific risk or protective factors, (d) did the parents or child have any specific physical or mental health problems, (e) what was the legal test used to render the court decision, and (f) what was the final ruling of the court. Generally, members determined the legal arguments made by judges when rendering foster care decisions and compared those arguments to the research in the areas of human development, marriage and family therapy, and family science.

During this meeting, a discussion ensued about the categories and themes. For example, the best interests of the child has traditionally been interpreted to mean protecting the welfare of the child or protecting children from unfit parents (Harvard Law Review (HLR), 1980; Pyle, 1994). To give another coding example, unlike criminal court cases, justices do not have to determine guilt beyond a reasonable doubt to terminate parental rights. Justices use the lower legal standard of clear and convincing evidence to terminate or protect parental rights. Clear and convincing evidence requires the facts presented make it highly probable that the claim is true; this standard has a greater burden than the preponderance of the evidence standard but it less rigorous than the standard of guilty beyond a reasonable doubt (Black et al., 1991). Students posed all legal questions to the faculty member with the family policy and law background to ensure accurate coding.

As seen in Table 2, there was an array of problems faced by the parents in the court cases reviewed by the cooperative research team, such as parental incarceration, or parental mental health issues that included but were not limited to substance abuse, bipolar disorders, schizophrenia, major depressive disorder, anxiety disorders, developmental disorders, or attention deficit/hyperactivity disorder. The rationale behind attending to mental health was based on the fact that the literature on foster care and parental rights rarely included the association of mental health issues and justices' decisions to terminate parental rights. Students pose questions about mental health issues to the faculty member with a marriage and family therapy background. Because of the diversity in the experiences of the parents in these cases, the content of the cases appealed to the interdisciplinary nature of family scholarship, e.g., family policy and law, marriage and family therapy, and family studies-and built on the unique and diverse experiences and/or expertise of members on the research team (Dinmore, 1997). Tables 1 and 2 were carefully reviewed and modified as deemed necessary, giving students the research questions to pose to the data, enhancing the trustworthiness of the data (Creswell, 1998; Strauss & Corbin, 1990).

In preparation for the second meeting and to ensure that everyone understood the material and coding schema, each team member was assigned one case to review and discuss at the second team meeting. Students were not to have any discussion about their case until the next meeting because we wanted to assess if the student understood the case. Furthermore, we wanted to asses their ability to code the case in a systematic and detailed manner and to examine the variability and consistency in their coding, referred to as trustworthiness in qualitative methods (Creswell, 1998; Strauss & Corbin, 1990).

## SECOND TEAM MEETING–PRELIMINARY CODING

At the second bi-weekly meeting, the team reassembled to review everyone's individual coding of the first case. The review lead to a discussion of coding discrepancies and ambiguities tended to fuel students curiosity. Critical debates about parental rights, children's rights, and the government's *parens patriae* powers used to protect the well-being of children or its police powers used to safeguard all citizens (Harvard Law Review, 1980) also were a result of the review and discussion processes. Students also questioned the new terms that emerged in the data, such as *ore tenus*, which refers to the presumption of accurateness that appellate courts give to the findings of fact reached by a trial court in a nonjury case (Black et al., 1991).

After this careful review process, we further developed a thematic coding structure for the project to include detailed instructions about the formatting of the data files. At this point, each member was assigned five court cases to code and was asked to compose an overview of information for each coded case. At this meeting, members also were paired off with a partner.

Using cooperative groups with paired teams, both group and individualized assignments were completed by students. One member of the paired team would code a case and send it to their partner to verify the categories, themes, and subthemes identified and to ensure consistency in and trustworthiness of the coding. This process continued throughout the semester until all five assigned cases were coded and verified. The partner system and extensive review of coding of court cases prepared the team to move into the actual implementation of Grounded Theory Methods (GTM). These interactions and team decisions set the parameters for all subsequent meetings.

Before closing the second meeting, faculty members wanted to further develop students' understanding of foster care policies. To put the coding of the foster care cases in context, we introduced the research team to three primary foster care policies, the Child Welfare Act of 1980 (CWA), Family Preservation and Support Services (FPSS) program, and Adoption and Safe Family Act (ASFA) (Adler, 2001; Administration of Children and Families, 1998, 2002, 2005; ARCH National Resource Center, 1994; Roberts, 2000). The cooperative research team also learned some family law history. For example, societal solutions used to promote the welfare of children, especially those in poorer families, included: (a) family dissolution and child placement in almshouses or orphanages in 1840s to 1850s, (b) family unification and child welfare by the 1860s, (c) family dissolution to reduce child maltreatment in the 1890s, and (d) family unification by providing mothers with child welfare services in the 1920s. Influenced by the *tender years doctrine*, in the 1920s children were viewed as citizens, instead of being parental property or the sole property of fathers. This shift in legal reasoning allowed justices to intrude upon parental rights to promote the welfare of children (Pyle, 1994). Later, child maltreatment or unfit parents legally justified the government's use of its *parens patriae* powers to intrude on the highly guarded rights of parents (Alder, 2001; HLR, 1980; Mnookin & Weisburg, 1993).

## *Subsequent Research Team Meetings: Grounded Theory Methods*

At subsequent research team meetings, we used GTM (Strauss & Corbin, 1990) to code the cases. Students used the thematic coding structure as a guide while they read the court cases and coded the content. As a reminder to readers, Table 1 provides students with the coding structure used by the cooperative research team. Beginning at the third meeting, the team met to discuss the first phase of GTM, termed open coding. During the open coding of court cases, team members continuously verified each other's work, ensuring continuity across the coding of the court cases, bringing any discrepancies that arose to the attention of all members during team meetings.

At each bi-weekly meeting, the GTM processes continued. Consequently, the next phase of the data analysis involved axial coding. In axial coding, a constant comparative method was used, where we went back and forth from the raw data and comparing it to the open coding, creating categories and connections in the data (Banks et al., 2000; Strauss & Corbin, 1990) that reflect the legal reasoning behind foster care decisions. In our axial coding of the data, we asked: (a) what evidence was presented to terminate parental rights (TPR), (b) how were developmental issues interpreted when justices upheld lower court decisions, and (c) what legal precedents did justices use to terminate the highly guarded rights of parents? Based on this process, we discovered themes that described the policies and legal evidence used to terminate parental rights. At this stage, one graduate student verified the axial coding prepared by all team members.

Here are some examples of the categories or themes students discovered, demonstrating their research competencies and understanding of foster care and family law. For instance, students correctly determined that children were placed in foster care due to allegations of child abuse or neglect, sexual assault, or because parents, usually those with substance abuse or other mental health issues, were deemed unfit. Termination of parental rights resulted if parents failed to strictly adhere to the foster care plan with little consideration given to the mental health issues of the parents, the absence of adequate transportation, or work skills. As seen in this direct quotation, the developmental concerns of parents (i.e., substance abuse, depression, developmental challenges, or schizophrenia) were noted, but exceptions were not likely to be made:

> *The trial court concluded that, although the evidence clearly supported termination of the mother's residual parental rights in all other respects, the mother's mental deficiency, which prevented her from properly caring for her child, constituted "good cause" under Code § 16.1-283(C)(2) for her inability to timely remedy the condition that led to the placement of her son in foster care. The Department contends the trial court erred in reaching that conclusion. We agree and reverse the trial court's judgment.* (Richmond Department of Social Services v. L. P., 2001, p. 1)

In fact, the court rulings that led to the termination of the highly guarded rights of parents were based on parents' failure to comply with the foster care plan. Parents were expected to: (a) maintain regular visits with the child, (b) complete parenting classes, (c) obtain employment, (d) comply with the assessment by the counselor, (e) attend the substance abuse treatment program, and/or (f) improve the conditions of the home environment. In *Barkey v. Commonwealth of VA, Alexandria Department of Social Services* (1986), for example, the parent was compliant but was characterized as being excessively tardy and failing to accept mental health and social support services. Ultimately, her parental rights were terminated in the Barkey case.

The final aspect of the data analysis was selective coding, using the coded data to develop a rich narrative that explains the phenomenon being studied. The selective coding of the data was the result of careful examination of the open and axial coding of the data. In this phase of the analysis, the goal is to fully explain all aspects of foster care decisions in Virginia; therefore, we questioned how justices' decisions and legal views reflect the socio-cultural context of foster care and parental rights and to determine under what circumstances did parents lose their parental rights. We also wanted to determine how the courts defined the best interests of the child to determine congruencies between social science indicators of healthy development from the vantage point of family science with the legal precedents that bind the hands of the courts. All coding and verification tasks were concluded before the last research team meeting. This type of project represents a unique experience for some students; some students did not have any previous research experience or a family law or policy background. Therefore, to effectively manage the cooperative group and to maintain realistic expectations for student learning, 30 of the 168 cases were coded during a 15-week semester.

## COOPERATIVE RESEARCH TEAM OUTCOMES

Besides coding and verifying the data, at the end of the semester, all students were required to submit personal narratives describing their reactions to both the content of the foster care cases they coded or verified, as well as the CL research team process. Depending upon the number of credit hours and individual student goals, some students completed a two-page critique of a peer-reviewed article using courts cases, wrote or modified an existing law to promote individual and family autonomy, or developed a one-page policy brief about foster care. Other students wrote a two-page court brief, identifying the plaintiff, respondent, facts of the case, legal reasoning, holding or conclusion, and dissenting or concurring opinion (for other ideas of cooperative learning activities see Cianciolo & Henderson, 2003; Cianciolo et al., 2001; Henderson & Martin, 2002).

As the end of the term neared, the research team met for a celebration. We spent the meeting sharing stories about the content we had read, talking about how far each member had advanced, and enjoyed the completion of a research endeavor. We gave each of the students a certificate of appreciation for their hard work and achievements. In addition to the expected results identified in the student objectives section of this manuscript, we learned that there were a number of unanticipated outcomes as well. One such outcome was that undergraduate and graduate students stated that they gained proficiency in the use of Word, Excel, and Power Point. Furthermore, students expressed that they felt compelled to continue in policy-related research. Additionally, the shared learning that occurred in research team meetings coupled with students' self-mastery of critical thinking, technological knowledge and research skills, produced very positive outcomes of the research experience. These endeavors, and the outcomes noted, support our university's research agenda for undergraduate students and demonstrate how our department has operationalized a supportive learning environment.

In general, all students demonstrated a growth in their understanding of family law in general and foster care policies more specifically. From the readings, handouts, and coding of the data, students were able to discuss how the lives of families were disrupted, regulated, and/or determined by judges and foster care laws. They were able to see a preliminary aggregation of the coded data and reflected on patterns that they saw, which to us, was confirmation of their learning. For instance, in all of the cases that were appealed after the implementation of ASFA resulted in the termination of parental rights. Students, in their reflection papers, noted this occurrence and provided opinions about the impact of the current policy on at-risk families.

Students also recognized that the developmental concerns of children were limited to the traditional definitions of child welfare–protecting children from harm or unfit parents. Thinking about their own family experiences, students noted that children from poor families were regulated more stringently than most middle- and upper-class families who were not expected to do everything perfectly. They were concerned about how family values were demonstrated by justices rendering foster care decisions. For example, In the *Barkey* case (1986), the court made this assertion:

> *The court must evaluate and consider many factors, including the age and physical and mental condition of the child or children; the age and physical and mental condition of the parents; the relationship existing between each parent and each child; the needs of the child or children; the role which each parent has played, and will play in the future, in the upbringing and care of the child or children; and such other factors.* (p. 4)

Despite this lengthy description, students noticed that the best interests of the child and the benefit to the parent-child relationship were not factored into the case. Their human development or family science training appeared incongruent with legal decision-making. They also recognized that ultimately courts determined that the best interests of the child was met through adoption (*Richmond Department of Social Services v. L.P.*, 2001) or terminating parental rights to provide children with a more permanent, stable adoptive home (for examples, see *Barkey v.*

*Commonwealth of VA, Alexandria Department of Social Services*, 1986; *Malave v. Fairfax County Department of Social Services*, 1999; *Richmond Department of Social Services v. L.P.*, 2001).

In other instances, students began asking questions about the intersection of poverty, neglect, policy, and the termination of parental rights. While current policy prohibits the removal of children because of poverty, there were cases where there seemed to be an association between social services definition of neglect and what members of the team coded as poverty. For example, evidence used to substantiate neglect included instances where there was "no electricity in the home," or a "broken window allowed mosquitoes to bite infant," or "children had head lice, were dirty and withdrawn." Because the students were able to see issues of poverty and neglect in context, their questions about the impact of current policy upon such families were informed by actual cases.

Another pattern that students noted was an association between mental health issues and termination of parental rights. Courts are to avoid making universal decisions regarding mental health and parental rights, but are instead mandated to consider whether or not the mental illness is "significantly detrimental" to parenting (Azar, Benjet, Fuhrmann, & Cavallero, 1995; Benjet, Azar, & Kuersten-Hogan, 2003). Yet, in every instance where a parent has a mental health issue presented to the courts post-Adoption and Safe Family Act, their parental rights were terminated. Non-compliance was a pervasive issue noted in the rationale provided to terminate parental rights. Thus, students began asking "how can social services better engage reluctant clients" and "can parents with mental health issues *really* demonstrate improvement in the conditions that lead to the removal of their children from the home within the timeframe mandated by ASFA?"

## *Undergraduate Outcomes*

As an assessment of the Cooperative Learning research team as a course, students completed a final evaluation. All of the undergraduate students ($n = 6$) rated the process as a 4.0 on a scale of 1.0 being lowest to 4.0 as highest. The most compelling indicator of students' learning occurred in their reflective commentaries about their growth and development. For instance, one students' anonymous written feedback illuminates the unexpected outcomes of CL:

> I feel this was far more useful than other courses I might have opted for in its place and I loved getting involved with this great experience... you have helped me figure out directions that I can go in the future and opened my eyes to a world I had no experience in.

In each of their narratives, students were able to explain their understanding of qualitative research, outline the growth in their research, team-building, and presentation skills, and explicate their knowledge of public policy and family law, including the fact that the law is legal, not moral.

Each of the undergraduate students involved in this process expressed an interest in attending graduate school, although all did not immediately apply. The literature speaks to a relationship between student retention rates and cooperative learning (Kluge, 1990; Totten et al., 1991), and the undergraduate outcomes in this instance provide tentative support for the influence of CL research teams on the recruitment of graduate students. The instructor-student relationship and the students' social skills were enhanced (Slavin, 1995b; Steven & Slavin, 1995) as a result of the research team experience.

One undergraduate student was responsible for showing a doctoral student research and administrative tasks for the research team. This student explained the coding schema and its purpose, gave a detailed overview of GTM, and shared why maintaining a journal is critical to the process of conducting qualitative research. The research expertise gained by this undergraduate student over a two-year period, a student who worked on research beyond the confines of a 15-week semester, demonstrates the effectiveness of allowing students to be active agents in their learning–another compelling indicator of learning and outcome of this innovative approach.

Some students presented the research as a poster at an undergraduate research symposium held annually at the university. Although the students reported that they were initially nervous about presenting, they reported a sense of pride in sharing their results with others. They learned how to create a research presentation and how to conduct themselves in a professional manner within an academic environment. They were able to build their resumes and professional experiences; we gave students ideas on how to note this research experience on their resume and letters of application to graduate school or for employment.

## Graduate Students

The graduate students on the CL research team gained experience with qualitative research, including GTM. The exposure to family law precedents and the constraints of the judicial system became an integral part of students' expertise and learning. Additionally, we gave them the option of writing a paper for publication and being part of a national conference, cultivating scholarly skills through presentations and manuscript preparations. Both students accepted this invitation. The Marriage and Family Therapy doctoral student is working on a paper to determine how justices addressed the termination of parental rights with parents with mental health concerns, whereas the Family Studies doctoral student is examining how justices define the best interests of the child when rendering foster care decisions. An abstract and submission of a scholarly manuscript are forthcoming for a national presentation.

## Faculty Outcomes

As the faculty members involved in this project, we have also benefited from this experience, which included managing a team that originally was housed on one campus to having duplicate data sets and files when one faculty member took a position in another state at the end of the academic year. As stated above, the CL experience is based on the premise that students and faculty are co-constructors of knowledge (Deering, 1989; Hertz-Lazarowitz & Shachar, 1990). Through this endeavor, we were able to conduct an investigation exploring the impact of policy upon families involved in the foster care system. We were able to present findings at national conferences and submit manuscripts for publication. Additionally, we were able to fine-tune our approaches to implementing cooperative research teams and transfer these lessons into our more traditional classroom teaching. For example, the faculty member who teaches family law and policy has recommitted herself to teaching students how to write a court brief, identifying the plaintiff, respondent, facts of the case, legal reasoning of the court, court ruling, dissent, and concurring opinions. The other faculty member, who teaches Marriage and Family Therapy, has integrated the study of policy into clinical courses.

In addition to the tangible outcomes we achieved, there were other intangible benefits as well. We very much enjoyed sharing our enthusiasm for a specific research topic with students. Watching students debate policy, become invested in the research project, and discover a passion for policy and research was invaluable to us as educators. Instead of feeling exhausted at the end of a semester, we were invigorated because of the CL research team experience.

## *CONCLUSION*

As a result of this project, students were engaged in a shared learning experience and were active agents of their learning (Dunlap & Grabinger, 1996; Johnson et al., 1991; Slavin & Cooper, 1999). Students were able to demonstrate improvements in their cognitive, social, and overall skills (Cohen & Lotan, 1997; Lotan & Whitcomb, 1998; Slavin, 1995a, 1995b; Stevens & Slavin, 1995), specifically in the areas of research, foster care policies, family law, written and oral communication proficiencies, and computer technologies. We found that self-management by students is a critical skill to learn, given that research fails to provide immediate rewards or outcomes. Lastly, we believe that using an interdisciplinary approach, integrating the research and theories in family policy and law, marriage and family therapy, family studies, and human development, benefited the research team. Given these advantages, cooperative learning may prove useful in courses on program development and evaluation, and parenting education and practice, helping students to put research to work and to simulate workforce experiences. The key to the success for Cooperative Learning is strategic planning and constant monitoring of students' work by faculty members.

Overall, cooperative research teams helped students understand how laws influence family development and families influence the law (Tanke & Tanke, 1979; Walters, 1983). Cooperative learning can result in improved individual and group achievement, and enhance students' critical thinking about family law and development. This pedagogical approach provided a mechanism for meeting the strategic goals of the department and university, but it also allowed students to direct their learning, enhance their overall skills, and gain some clarity and direction for their immediate and distant professional endeavors. Additionally, the faculty members were able to use their teaching expertise and knowledge to support their scholarship. The collegial relationship between the faculty members gives some evidence about how CL improves the social development of the instructors, not just the students. Ultimately, we believe that Cooperative Learning research teams are an innovative and effective way to teach family law, and it is a productive way to use our human capital resources in economically lean times that confront institutions of higher learning.

# REFERENCES

Adoption and Safe Families Act (ASFA), Public Law 105-89. (1997).
Adler, L. S. (2001). The meanings of permanence: A critical analysis of the Adoption and Safe Family Act of 1997. Retrieved on May 10, 2003, from *http://web.lexis.com*
Administration for Children and Families. (1998). Program instructions: New legislation–public law 105-89, the Adoption and Safe Families Act of 1997 Retrieved on March 30, 2005 from *www.acf.hhs.gov/programs/cb/laws/pi/pi9802.htm*
Administration for Children and Families. (2002). National foster care and adoption information: Data collection systems. Retrieved on March 8, 2005 from *http://www.acf.dhhs.gov/programs/cb/dis/tables/sec11gb/national.htm*
Administration for Children and Families. (2005). National adoption and foster care statistics. Retrieved on March 8, 2005, from *http://www.acf.hhs.gov/programs/cb/dis/afcars/publications/afcars.htm*.
Anderson, E. A. & Skinner, D. A. (1995). The components of family policy education. *Journal of Family and Economics Issue, 16*, 65-77.
ARCH National Resource Center. (1994). *Family Preservation and Family Support Services: ARCH Factsheet Number 37*. Retrieved on April 25, 2003, from *http://www.chtop.com/ARCH/archfs37.htm*
Azar, S. T., Benjet, C. L., Fuhrmann, G. S., & Cavallero, L. (1995). Child maltreatment and termination of parental rights: Can behavioral research help Solomon? *Behavior Therapy, 26*, 599-623.
Banks, S. P., Louie, E., & Einerson, M. (2000). Constructing personal identities in holiday letters. *Journal of Social and Personal Relationships, 17*, 299-327.
Barkey v. Commonwealth of VA, Alexandria Department of Social Services. (1986). App. LEXIS 0290-85. Retrieved on December 21, 2002, from http://web.lexis-nexis.com
Benjet, C., Azar, S. T., & Kuersten-Hogan, R. (2003) Evaluating the parental fitness of psychiatrically diagnosed individuals: Advocating a functional-contextual analysis of parenting. *Journal of Family Psychology, 17*, 238-251.
Black, H. C., Nolan, J. R., & Nolan-Haley, J. M. (1991). *Black's Law Dictionary*. St. Paul. MN: West.
Child Welfare Act. 42 U.S.C.A. §§ 670. (1980).
Cianciolo, P., Henderson, T., Kretzer, S., & Mendes, A. (2001). Promoting collaborative learning strategies in aging and public policy courses. *Gerontology and Geriatrics Education, 22*, 47-67.
Cianciolo, P. & Henderson, T. (2003). Infusing aging and public policy content into gerontology courses: Collaborative learning methods to teach about social security and Medicare. *Educational Gerontology, 29*, 217-233.
Cohen, E. G. & Lotan, R. A. (1997). *Working for equality in heterogeneous classrooms: Sociological theory in practice*. New York: Teachers College Press.
Creswell, J. W. (1998). *Qualitative inquiry and research design: Choosing among five traditions*. Thousand Oaks, CA: Sage.
Deering, P. D. (1989, October). An ethnographic approach for examining participants' construction of a cooperative learning class culture. Paper presented at the annual

meeting of the American Anthropological Association, Washington, DC. (ERIC Document Reproduction Service No. ED 319 083).

Dinmore, I. (1997). Interdisciplinary and integrative learning: An imperative for adult education. Retrieved on October 6, 2000, from Dow Jones Interactive Database.

Dunlap, J. C. & Grabinger, R. S. (1996). Rich environments for active learning in the higher education classroom. In B. G. Wilson (Ed.), *Constructivist learning environments: Case studies in instructional design* (pp. 65-82). Englewood Cliffs, NJ: Educational Technologies Publications.

Family Preservation and Support Services, Omnibus Budget Reconciliation Act of 1993, P. L. 103-66P. (1993).

Goodwin, M. W. (1999). Cooperative learning and social skills: What skills to teach and how to teach them. *Intervention in School and Clinic, 35*, 29-33.

*Harvard Law Review.* (1980). Developments in the law: The Constitution and the family. Boston, MA: Author.

Henderson, T. L. & Martin, K. (2002). Cooperative learning as one approach to teaching family law. *Family Law, 51*, 351-360.

Hertz-Lazarowitz, R. & Shachar, H. (1990). Teacher's verbal behavior in cooperative and whole class instruction. In S. Sharan (Ed.) *Cooperative learning: Theory and research* (pp. 77-94). New York: Praeger.

Johnson, D. W., Johnson, R. T., Holubec, E. J., & Roy, P. (1994). *Circles of learning: Cooperation in the classroom.* Alexandria, VA: The Association for Supervision and Curriculum Development.

Johnson, D. W., Johnson, R. T., & Smith, K. (1991). *Active learning: Cooperation in the college classroom.* Edina, MN: Interaction.

Kluge, L. (1990). *Cooperative learning.* Arlington, VA: Educational Research Service.

Lotan, R. A. & Whitcomb, J. A. (1998). *Group work in diverse classrooms.* New York: Teachers College Press.

*Malave v. Fairfax County Department of Social Services.* (1999). App. LEXIS 2708-98-4. Retrieved on December 21, 2002, from *http://web.lexis-nexis.com*

Mnookin, R. H., & Weisburg, D. K. (1993). *Child, family, and state: Problems and materials on children and law* (2nd ed.). Boston, MA: Little, Brown and Company.

*Moore v. the City of East Cleveland,* 431 U.S. 494; 97 S. Ct. 1932; 1977 U.S. LEXIS 17; 52 L. Ed. 2d 531.

Nolinske, T. & Millis, B. (1997). Cooperative learning as an approach to pedagogy. *The American Journal of Occupational Therapy, 53*, 31-40.

Pyle, R. C. (1994). *Family law.* Albany, NY: Delmar.

*Richmond Department of Social Services v. L.P.* (2001). App. LEXIS 1737-00-2. Retrieved on December 21, 2002, from *http://web.lexis-nexis.com*

Roberts, D. E. (2000). *Is there justice in children's rights? The critique of federal family preservation policy.* Retrieved on September 30, 2002, from *http://www. law.upenn.edu/conlaw/vol2/num1/roberts_ct.html*

Slavin, R. E. (1995a). *Cooperative learning: Theory, research, and practice* (2nd ed.). Boston: Allyn & Bacon.

Slavin, R. E. (1995b). Cooperative learning and intergroup relations. In J. Banks and C. M. Banks (Eds.), *Handbook of research on multicultural education* (pp. 628-634). New York: Macmillan.

Slavin, R. E. & Cooper, R. (1999). Improving intergroup relations: Lessons learned from cooperative learning programs. *Journal of Social Issues, 55*, 647-663.

Steiner, S., Stromwell, K. L., Brzuzy, S., & Gerdes, K. (1999). Using cooperative learning strategies in social work education. *Journal of Social Work Education, 35*, 253-264.

Stevens, R. J. & Slavin, R. E. (1995). The cooperative elementary school: Effects on students' achievement, attitudes, and social relations. *American Educational Research Journal, 32*, 321-351.

Stodolsky, S. S. (1984). Frameworks for studying instructional processes in peer work-groups. In P. L. Peterson, L. C. Wilkinson, & M. Hallinan (Eds.), *Group organization and group processes* (pp. 107-124). Orlando, FL: Academic Press.

Strauss, A. & Corbin, J. (1990). *Basics of qualitative research: Grounded theory procedures and techniques*. Newbury Park, CA: Sage.

Tanke, E, D. & Tanke, T. J. (1979). Getting off a slippery slope: Social science in the judicial process. *American Psychologist, 34*, 1130-1138.

Totten, S., Sills, T., & Digby, A. (1991). *Cooperative learning: A guide to research*. New York: Garland.

Walker, A. J. (1996). Cooperative learning in the classroom. *Family Relations, 45*, 521-526.

Walters, L. H. (1983). The role of family specialists and research in the law. *Family Relations, 32*, 521-526.

# An Exploratory Examination of Students' Family Policy Beliefs

Randy Leite
Ruben P. Viramontez Anguiano

**ABSTRACT.** Family policy is coming to be recognized as an important component of programs focusing on family issues. As political leaders continue to engage in debates about family issues and family service professionals report spending more time on policy issues within their professional practice, attention to policy issues has become more important in the education of students in family courses. Because of the increasing presence of public policy study within the family studies curricula, it is important to consider students' policy perceptions and experiences as they enter family policy classes. Argued here is that students are more likely to become engaged with family policy topics that are timely and meaningful to them. This research examines student perceptions of various policy topics and issues in an attempt to better design courses with family policy content. *[Article copies available for a fee from The Haworth Document Delivery Service: 1-800-HAWORTH. E-mail address: <docdelivery@haworthpress.com> Website: <http://www.HaworthPress.com> © 2005 by The Haworth Press, Inc. All rights reserved.]*

**KEYWORDS.** Family policy, policy, student perceptions, teaching

---

Randy Leite and Ruben P. Viramontez Anguiano are affliated with Bowling Green State University.

Address correspondence to: Randy Leite, Human Development and Family Studies Program, 206 Johnston Hall, Bowling Green State University, Bowling Green, OH 43403 (E-mail: rleite@bgnet.bgsu.edu).

The authors would like to thank Jessica Theis and Jacqueline Walter, both graduate students in the Human Development and Family Studies program at Bowling Green State University, for their assistance with this research.

## INTRODUCTION

Public policy, as an organized field of study, has existed since the early years of the twentieth century (Laswell, 1951). In many ways, however, policy studies is still in a developmental stage (Nagel, 1999). In fact, within this long history of attention to public policy, there has been relatively little attention to family policy. This deficit is reflected in the ongoing lack of consensus among policy scholars as to a basic definition of the term "family policy" (Bogenschneider, 2002). Kamerman and Kahn (1978) suggested that family policy is any government action that affects families. Zimmerman (1995) refined this definition and suggested that family policy constitutes a collection of separate but interrelated policy choices that aim to address problems that families experience. Moen and Schorr (1987) focus on the objectives of family policy rather than its source or structure and define family policy as a "widely agreed-on set of objectives for families toward the realization of which the state deliberately shapes programs or policies" (p. 4).

This deficit is also reflected in the lack of degree programs preparing family specialists which address family policy. A review of 100 undergraduate family science programs in the United States indicates that slightly over half currently include a course in family policy and/or family law, while several others include courses from other disciplines such as sociology or political science that specifically address family policy or include family policy within broad attention to social policy. Moreover, attention to family policy in curricula addressing family issues is further complicated when the context of culture is included in the discussion of family policy.

Although family and cultural diversity courses are becoming more common in programs that have family courses (Viramontez Anguiano & Harrison, 2002), the interface between the two demands more attention from scholars (Lerner, Sparks, & McCubbin, 1999; McAdoo, 1999). This deficiency has not only created a void in curricula, but also a workforce of family professionals who have little or no training in culturally sensitive family policy.

Clearly, family is often at the center of debates on controversial issues. On any given day, news outlets are filled with reports of the debates that rage over issues such as the definition of marriage, family-based benefit programs, education and family services funding, and other family policy issues, including Medicare, welfare reform, and marriage promotion programs. Because of advances in media and technology, U.S. citizens are exposed to debates on these issues more frequently than in previous eras. This is especially true for undergraduate students who are typically consumers of various media, including television, online news sources, weblogs and discussion forums. All provide information that might influence student beliefs about various policy issues.

Ongoing trends in American family life (e.g., increased use of reproductive technology, increased number of working parents) provide a further justification for exploring the status of public policy within programs preparing family professionals (de Leon & Steelman, 2000). Media discussions of controversial family issues (i.e., welfare reform, same sex marriage) often include attention to policy topics and concerns. In light of the fact that policy issues and decisions are becoming even more visible in American family life, it is imperative that family policy be included in programs addressing family life and family issues.

While most students do not enter family-focused programs with a strong interest in policy or the policy process, it is a content area that is proving to be of greater importance as they graduate and enter their respective professions. Indeed, family service professionals report that attention to public policy should be a critical component in the preparation of students entering the field (Leite & Landry Meyer, 2003).

Thus, policy is central to the work of family professionals such as family life educators, social service workers, child and family case workers, family counselors, agency administrators, family scholars, family attorneys, family advocates, and others who may play a role in the development, enactment, implementation, or assessment of social policies (Bogenschneider, 2002; Keller, Whittaker, & Burke, 2001). This requires engagement with political processes that exist at all levels of policymaking. It has been suggested that few students show a strong desire to understand or participate in politics because they lack either the resources or the knowledge to do so (Verba, Schlozman, & Brady, 1995). While these may not be the only factors contributing to this pattern of disengagement, it is clearly important to develop such resources and knowledge among students preparing to enter human services careers.

A perspective on how to facilitate this development may be drawn from Kingsdon's (1995) concept of policy windows. Kingsdon suggested that researchers who wish to influence policy decisions may more effectively do so by focusing on topics that are presently relevant for policymakers. Such relevance may be determined by the degree to which issues are addressed in the media, generate interest among the electorate, or hold meaning in the lives of political constituents. Much as a window opens and closes, Kingsdon suggests opportunities to impact policymakers open and close based on fluctuations in relevance or meaning of various topics.

Although students develop interest s in policy issues for very different reasons than legislators, Kingsdon's basic view may still be applied to assessing teachable moments relating to policy in programs addressing family issues. Such teachable moments may be viewed as the windows of opportunity during which students may be more likely to take an interest in particular policy topics. These opportunities may be created by significant public attention to, and media portrayals of, policy issues, or when a student is personally impacted by a policy issue. At these times, students take notice of issues that may also be highly relevant to their later work as family professionals. This heightened interest offers an opportunity for instructors to utilize attention to those topics as avenues to explore the policy process and other important policy topics of which students may be less aware. Thus, as Kingsdon argues in relation to policymakers, it is important for those teaching family policy courses to discover those topics that may resonate with students at a particular time.

The present study is an exploration of potential open policy windows among today's students. Specifically, the purpose of this exploratory study was to develop a better understanding of students' perceptions of family policy and family policy issues. Students at two large Midwestern universities were asked their perspectives on a variety of policy topics and their assessments of the importance of potential policy course content areas. Special attention was given to the issue of policy's relationship to promoting cultural sensitivity and understanding of cultural diversity and also to students' awareness of the political leaders who represent them.

## METHOD

Two hundred and ten undergraduate students were surveyed in human development and family studies courses at two large Midwestern universities. These included students enrolled both in entry-level and upper-level family science undergraduate courses. None of the undergraduate students had taken a family policy class nor had family policy been discussed in their present classes prior to the administration of the survey instrument. A demographic profile of the student sample is provided in Table 1. The sample largely reflects the distribution of students

TABLE 1. Sample Demographics

| Demographic Factor | Number (%) |
|---|---|
| **Class Year** | |
| Freshman | 79 (37.6%) |
| Sophomore | 42 (20.0%) |
| Junior | 48 (22.9%) |
| Senior | 41 (19.5%) |
| **Sex** | |
| Female | 181 (86.2%) |
| Male | 29 (13.8%) |
| **Race** | |
| Caucasian | 183 (87.1%) |
| African-American | 11 (5.2%) |
| Hispanic | 6 (2.9%) |
| Other | 5 (2.5%) |
| **Age** | |
| Mean | 20.74 years |
| Std. Dev. | 4.30 years |

in classes at institutions across the United States in that it is largely female, Caucasian, and is comprised of students whose average age is approximately 21.

Students were asked to complete a survey addressing family policy issues. The survey included both quantitative and qualitative items. Respondents were asked to provide their own definition of "family policy," and to identify up to three family policy issues they believed were important in their localities. Respondents were also asked to indicate whether or not they would characterize each of fourteen items as being significant family policy issues in the United States. These included defense of marriage policy, welfare reform, education funding, divorce law, social security, nutrition policy, employment policy, reduction of juvenile delinquency, marriage promotion policy, child custody, health care policy, Medicare, educational reform policy, and policy regarding same-sex unions.

To assess knowledge of actors in state and federal policymaking processes, students were also asked to name one of their representatives to the state legislature (either their state senator or their state representative), their United States Representative, and one of their United States

Senators. While not directly addressing policy issues, this information was indicative of student awareness of state and federal politics.

Students were also asked to address issues of content in family policy courses. Using a ten-point scale ranging from 10-"very important" to 1-"not important," students rated the importance of including each of fifteen possible areas of content in a family policy class. These included historical policy perspectives, current family trends, levels of policy and policymaking, the policymaking process, links between research and policy, family impact analysis, family theory frameworks and their relation to policy, family policy frameworks, advocacy and education roles in the policy process, roles for family service professionals in the policy process, and five general areas of policy formation: poverty/welfare policy, marriage policy, child custody policy, work-family policy, and education reform policy.

Finally, respondents were asked to provide comments in response to qualitative prompts concerning what is important when developing culturally sensitive family policy. These included items that focused on important factors and attributes associated with culturally-sensitive family policy and strengths of diverse families that might serve to inform public policy. Specifically, students were asked qualitative semi-structured questions that addressed factors associated with culturally-sensitive family policy, important attributes of programs that serve diverse families, and strengths of diverse families that might inform family policy.

Data were analyzed through a variety of statistical and qualitative techniques. Policy definitions and student responses to the cultural sensitivity items were assessed through a process of theme analysis in which recurring themes were extracted from the student responses (Miles & Huberman, 1994). In all cases, responses were read and themes identified by two raters based on guiding categories. Frequencies were calculated for students' identification of topics as significant policy issues and explorations of any correlation between these ratings and various demographic factors were conducted, using the contingency correlation coefficient. A one-way analysis of variance was conducted in relation to students' assessment of the importance of various areas of possible course content.

## *RESULTS*

Students were initially asked to define family policy. It is clear that undergraduate student definitions of family policy are far-ranging and often ambiguous. However, student responses generally fit into one of three categories. The first of these are broad definitions offering few limitations on what might be considered family policy, how policy is formed, or by whom. These include definitions such as, "anything dealing with family life," "policies that benefit families" and "legislation that affects the family." These definitions are so broad as to reflect little meaningful understanding of the scope of family policy. The second category of definitions are those focusing on impacts on specific areas of family life including specific aspects of family structure and functioning or focused on specific categories of issues. Many of these comments included such factors as promoting family well-being, offering support to families, contributing to family cohesion, and impacts on family structure. Examples of such definitional statements include "policies that make a well-rounded and constructed family," "a policy that states important aspects of a family," and "anything that promotes the structure and well-being of families." These definitions largely reflect a perspective that suggests family policy is developed by government or other representative bodies for the benefit of families. Finally, many students perceived family policy as being an aspect of families themselves. These definitions largely reflected the concept of family policy as consisting of rules, patterns, or responses within families that either contribute to family functioning or guide members' behaviors. In this area, examples of student responses include, "something having to do with what a family values," "a family's morals," "a plan within a family on how they carry out daily routines," and "rules that are decided within the family and that the family agrees to follow." This perspective is substantially different from the others in that it reflects no concept of policy as existing on a larger social level and as being developed outside families.

The second qualitative piece of this exploratory study concerned student perceptions regarding the possible link between family policy and development of cultural sensitivity and diversity. Three categories were utilized to examine the data through a theme analysis: culturally sensitive family policy, effective programs and the strengths of diverse families (Lerner et al., 1999; McAdoo, 1999; Rotter & Casado, 1998). Generally, students focused on degrees and aspects of cultural sensitivity in family policy (i.e., "Policies should address the issues of families in different cultural groups."), issues concerning the effectiveness of programs in promoting understanding of cultural issues (i.e., "It would be good for programs to train their staff in diversity issues."), and programmatic attention to and utilization of perceived strengths of diverse families (i.e., "Families from different groups have different strengths that should be included in policies.").

Students also were asked to identify three significant family policy issues in their localities. As indicated in Table 2, a wide variety of issues were generated with no single issue being identified by more than a third of all respondents. Education, poverty/welfare, marriage/divorce, child custody, and health care policies were most frequently mentioned, with 42 issues being mentioned by at least one student. A total of 68 (32.4%) respondents did not list a single issue as being significant in their locality.

Beyond these local issues, students were also asked to identify significant policy issues at the national level. They were presented with a list of fourteen items commonly mentioned by political leaders in discussing family issues. A further exploration of these responses was con-

TABLE 2. Local Policy Issues Identified by Students (Number and Percent)

| Issue | Number (%) |
|---|---|
| Education | 69 (32.9%) |
| Poverty/Welfare Policy | 52 (24.8%) |
| Marriage/Divorce | 32 (15.2%) |
| Health Care | 30 (14.3%) |
| Child Custody | 28 (13.3%) |
| Employment | 19 (9.1%) |
| Same-Sex Marriage | 16 (7.6%) |
| Abuse/Domestic Violence | 15 (7.1%) |
| Social Security | 14 (6.7%) |
| IDEA | 14 (6.7%) |
| No Child Left Behind | 13 (6.2%) |
| Taxes | 11 (5.2%) |
| Medicare | 10 (4.8%) |
| Child Support | 9 (4.3%) |
| Neglect | 7 (3.3%) |
| Family Involvement | 6 (2.9%) |
| Adoption | 6 (2.9%) |
| Abortion | 6 (2.9%) |
| Food | 5 (2.4%) |
| Child Care | 5 (2.4%) |

22 issues mentioned by 3 or fewer respondents

ducted in relation to four demographic variables: student age, race, sex, and class year to determine if any of these items contributed to variations in student responses. The number of students specifying each topic as important and correlations among demographic variables and the various policy topics are summarized in Table 3.

As indicated, few relationships were found between the assessed demographic variables and student characterizations of the fourteen topic areas as significant family policy issues. Females were more likely to report divorce law higher in importance than did males. Education issues (educational funding and education reform) were more likely to be reported as significant by students in later class years than among students in earlier class years. Older students were also more likely to label educational funding as an important issue than younger students. Student race was not associated with variations in student responses on any of the fourteen topics, perhaps reflecting the largely racially homogeneous sample.

An effort was also made to determine the degree to which students are aware of the political leaders who represent them in the policymaking process. Relatively few students could name their state senator or repre-

TABLE 3. Students Identifying Topics as Significant Policy Issues (Contingency Correlation Coefficient)

| Issue | Number (%) | Sex (df = 1) | Class Year (df = 3) | Race (df = 3) | Age (df = 1) |
|---|---|---|---|---|---|
| Defense of Marriage | 126 (60.0%) | .835 | .098 | .999 | .910 |
| Welfare Reform | 81 (38.6%) | .148 | .194 | .090 | .523 |
| Education Funding | 72 (34.3%) | .476 | .044* | .742 | .039* |
| Divorce Law | 104 (49.5%) | .050* | .978 | .953 | .126 |
| Social Security | 114 (54.3%) | .777 | .734 | .793 | .236 |
| Nutrition Policy | 112 (53.3%) | .693 | .707 | .900 | .793 |
| Employment Policy | 102 (48.6%) | .573 | .062 | .377 | .106 |
| Reducing Juvenile Delinquency | 109 (51.9%) | .799 | .470 | .404 | .606 |
| Marriage Promotion | 128 (61.0%) | .908 | .117 | .370 | .088 |
| Child Custody | 70 (33.3%) | .209 | .031 | .264 | .087 |
| Health Care | 74 (35.2%) | .068 | .112 | .337 | .193 |
| Medicare | 115 (54.8%) | .336 | .372 | .265 | .680 |
| Education Reform | 85 (40.5%) | .731 | .002* | .792 | .092 |
| Same-Sex Marriage | 129 (61.4%) | .862 | .025 | .637 | .124 |

* $p < .05$

sentative, United States representative, and one United States senator who represent their home district. Only 30 (14.3%) of the respondents could correctly identify one of their state legislators, 36 (17.1%) could correctly identify one of their United States Senators, and only 28 (13.3%) could correctly identify their U.S. Representative. There was no significant variation in responses.

Finally, students were asked to identify the importance of particular areas of course content in a family policy class. Students were presented with a list of fifteen course topics and asked to rate their importance on a ten-point scale, ranging from 10-Very Important to 1-Not Important. Table 4 provides mean responses for undergraduate students and indicators of association with four demographic variables: student age, race, sex, and class year.

As was the case with the importance students ascribed to various national policy issues, few relationships were found between the demographic variables and ratings of course topics. Gender was associated with the importance assigned to historical perspectives, family theory, and family policy frameworks, with males all viewing them as more im-

TABLE 4. Student Assessment of Importance of Possible Course Content (One-Way Analysis of Variance)

| Content Area | Mean (SD) | Sex (df =1) | Class Year (df = 3) | Race (df = 3) | Age (df = 1) |
|---|---|---|---|---|---|
| Historical Perspectives | 6.23 (2.01) | .000* | .003* | .454 | .276 |
| Family Trends | 8.10 (1.63) | .802 | .734 | .956 | .829 |
| Levels of Policy | 7.07 (1.83) | .595 | .424 | .857 | .928 |
| Policy Process | 7.02 (1.88) | .498 | .888 | .329 | .799 |
| Links between Research & Policy | 7.09 (5.31) | .237 | .525 | .843 | .840 |
| Family Impact Analysis | 7.88 (1.73) | .357 | .839 | .767 | .198 |
| Family Theory Frameworks | 7.28 (1.85) | .039* | .845 | .928 | .478 |
| Family Policy Frameworks | 7.48 (1.86) | .028* | .695 | .604 | .716 |
| Policy Advocacy vs. Policy Education | 7.65 (1.59) | .555 | .452 | .814 | .650 |
| Professional Roles | 7.57 (1.52) | .412 | .987 | .173 | .591 |
| Poverty/Welfare Reform Policy | 7.83 (1.83) | .579 | .681 | .077 | .476 |
| Marriage/Marriage Promotion Policy | 7.74 (1.93) | .820 | .809 | .049* | .799 |
| Work-Family Policy | 8.44 (1.50) | .803 | .799 | .795 | .131 |
| Education Policy | 9.30 (1.07) | .350 | .026* | .447 | .052 |
| Child Custody Policy | 8.48 (1.61) | .083 | .361 | .899 | .936 |

* $p < .05$

portant than females. Student class year was associated with greater importance ascribed to historical perspectives and education policy, with students in later class years rating them higher than students in earlier class years. Caucasian students were more likely to identify marriage and marriage promotion programs as being important than other racial groups. Student age was not significantly associated with variation in response to any of the topics.

## *DISCUSSION*

The purpose of this exploratory study was to develop a better picture of undergraduate students' perceptions of family policy issues. With greater attention to such issues in undergraduate curricula and increased calls for programs to better prepare graduates for positions in family service administration (Kearns, 1998; Nagel, 1999), such insights are of value to those who teach family policy courses. These data offer a number of insights regarding policy topics that might generate more interest among students and provide instructors with an opportunity to expand teaching and learning activities.

These results provide a number of insights regarding students' perceptions and preferences concerning family policy. Chief among these is the obvious fact that students have little understanding of what constitutes family policy. Over 160 definitions of family policy were provided by students with considerable variation among them. It is clear many students do not understand that family policy is formulated outside of families. Nor are they aware of the primary sources of family policy. Such a lack of understanding is consistent with students' relatively low level of engagement with policy processes and political issues.

Because of a major deficiency in students' fundamental understanding of family policy as a concept, it is important this topic be addressed within curricula and courses focusing on family issues. Students should be challenged to not only consider policy definitions, but to continuously examine those definitions associated with family policy. These data suggest that instructors should focus on the definition of family policy as a useful starting point in undergraduate family policy classes.

Student confusion regarding definitions of family policy is further evident in the variation that exists in their identification of family policy topics that are relevant in their localities. Nearly one-third of all respondents were unable to identify even a single issue as important. Among those who did identify topics as being locally important, a wide variety of issues were identified, with poverty/welfare policy, marriage/divorce, health care, child custody, and education being mentioned most frequently. This suggests that these topics may hold more relevance among students.

Similar insight may be drawn from student characterizations of various family policy topics as important. Not surprisingly, the most commonly-identified family policy topics are four that have received considerable media attention over the past year: same-sex unions, marriage promotion, defense of marriage, and Medicare. It is not clear as to what degree students distinguish differences among the three of these that relate to aspects of marriage or whether they define these as all being a part of marriage policy. While policy relating to same-sex unions is generally viewed as addressing relationships more broadly than within the legal status of marriage (i.e., domestic partner benefits, survivor benefits, etc.), marriage promotion policy focuses on encouraging marriage among at-risk populations. The defense of marriage initiatives are viewed as an attempt to define marriage as strictly between a male and a female. But such distinctions may not be clear to students.

All four of the topics most frequently identified by students have been the subject of extensive debate over the past year and this may be viewed as contributing to student awareness of these issues. Moreover, this reinforces the notion that the mass media is an important educational mechanism (Levine, 1998). Specifically, the mass media provides a window of opportunity for exposing the students to controversial family policy issues. While these issues do not necessarily coincide with the most frequently-mentioned issues of importance in student localities, the data reflect the responses of the entire student sample rather than a subset of students who identified one or more local issues.

Respondents were more likely to identify topics receiving considerable media attention as important policy issues. This suggests that such issues may generate greater interest among students and also serve as avenues for introducing various course topics. If viewed as opportunities to create teachable moments, these highly rated issues should be built into family curricula in an effort to promote student learning of family policy concepts. Therefore, it is argued that student learning is enhanced when family policy courses incorporate timely and relevant policy issues into class discussions or are included in demonstrations of course concepts.

The data regarding respondent assessment of the importance of various family policy course topics also offers useful insights. Topics that included specific family policy issues were viewed by students as most important. As indicated in Table 4, these include education reform policy, child custody policy, and welfare policy. This is not surprising in light of student indications and ratings of important issues as reflected in Tables 2 and 3. While it may be argued that educational reform is not family policy, this issue has received considerable attention in the state in which these data were collected and has frequently been presented as benefiting children and families. This may account for the degree to which students identified it as an important family policy issue.

Also, and perhaps not surprisingly, students listed as least important such topics as historical perspectives, the policy process, and policy formulation. This offers further support for the policy windows perspective in that the data suggests greater student interest in and assessment of the importance of topical policy issues. This is not to suggest that only those topics of interest to students should be included in a family policy course. Rather, topics that interest students most should be used more frequently as vehicles for introducing them to the policymaking process.

The qualitative findings demonstrated that students have begun to develop a basic knowledge of the interface between cultural sensitivity and family policy. In addition, students demonstrated a belief that cultural sensitivity should center on family strengths. Their responses also reflected an understanding of the importance of addressing family policy through multiple factors, including ethnic and cultural differences, socioeconomic status and educational disparities. A possible explanation for these findings is that students in family-focused programs are being exposed to cultural diversity and cultural sensitivity throughout their college careers. Moreover, family and cultural diversity courses are becoming more common in the field of human development and family studies. As a result, students in the field may have a greater awareness of diversity issues. Therefore, the category addressing strengths of diverse families and its three themes should be considered a critical component of family policy education.

A related thematic category, effective programming, suggests students were beginning to incorporate knowledge about culturally sensitive practice into an understanding of family policy. Specifically, the students reflected a belief that different dimensions of diversity are important in the creation of family policy. Such findings imply that cultural diversity issues may be effectively incorporated into family policy courses. Further, family policy course content might be effectively linked with family diversity course content to promote the students' critical understandings in each area.

The qualitative findings demonstrate the students' understanding of the importance of addressing ethnic and cultural differences, socioeconomic status and educational disparities in formulating and implementing family policy. The responses further suggest that undergraduate students are gaining an appreciation for family and cultural diversity and an understanding of the importance of the interface between cultural diversity and family policy. One explanation for this growth is that human development and family studies students and other students in the helping professions are being exposed to more culturally sensitive material throughout their college careers. Therefore, as family and cultural diversity courses become more common in the field of human development and family studies, students are more likely to develop a greater awareness of diversity issues in relation to their chosen professions.

## RECOMMENDATIONS FOR INSTRUCTORS

A number of recommendations for instructors of family policy courses may be drawn from this research. First, instructors incorporating policy into family curricula should consider explaining the policy process through the use of topical class presentations by seizing the teachable moment and discussing issues to which students can easily relate. Process issues associated with policy formation, implementation, and evaluation may be more effectively addressed if subject areas that hold relevance and meaning to students are built into instructional content.

Second, it is important that instructors not focus exclusively on the topics that generate the highest level of awareness or interest among students. In preparing human services professionals, it is important that faculty address a wide range of policy issues that may be particularly relevant to students on various career paths. To this end, instructors should explore strategies for incorporating important but less recognized areas of public policy into courses.

Third, faculty need to be more effective in exploring ways to link selected policy issues with topics that generate more interest among students. For example, attention to policies concerning adoption rights of same-sex partners might be channeled first through a discussion of second-parent adoption and then on to a discussion of adoption policy in general. Similarly, a general discussion of child custody policy might be expanded into a discussion of visitation policy, paternity policy, and child support enforcement policy.

Fourth, instructors should take time during a class session early in the term to survey students with respect to their interest in current events and their understanding of the political system. The information gathered should prove useful in developing course content and preparing class lectures on various policy topics. Such information should be shared with other colleagues through published journal articles and presentations at professional conferences.

Finally, while family policy courses should not be political science courses, it would be useful for instructors to build into their course syllabi appropriate material that explains the political structure and the policy process. Concurrently, students should be encouraged to develop a greater understanding of the policymaking process and be able to identify key political actors in their own localities. It is reasonable to assume that instructors will seek and find appropriate teachable moments and exploit them accordingly.

Clearly, in light of the numerous family policy debates being undertaken among political leaders and family service professionals, family policy will continue to grow in importance as a topic to be addressed in family programs. Faculty must develop an arsenal of strategies to better integrate policy content into curricula. The recommendations contained herein offer a start in that direction.

## REFERENCES

Bogenschneider, K. (2002). *Family policy matters: How policymaking affects families and what professionals can do.* Mahweh, NJ: Lawrence Erlbaum Associates.

de Leon, P. & Steelman, T.A. (2000). Making public policy programs effective and relevant: The role of the policy sciences. *Journal of Public Policy Analysis and Management, 20,* 163-171.

Kamerman, S. B. & Kahn, A. J. (1978). Families and the idea of family policy. In S.B. Kamerman & A.J. Kahn (Eds.), *Family policy: Government and families in fourteen countries* (pp. 1-16). New York: Columbia University Press.

Keller, T. E., Whittaker, J. K., & Burke, T. K. (2001). Student debates in policy courses: Promoting policy practice skills and knowledge through active learning. *Journal of Social Work Education, 37,* 343-355.

Kearns, K. P. (1998). Institutional accountability in higher education: A strategic approach. *Public Productivity and Management Review, 22,* 140-156.

Kingsdon, J.W. (1995). *Agendas, alternatives, and public policies.* New York: HarperCollins.

Laswell, H. (1951). The policy orientation. In D. Lerner & H. Laswell (Eds.), *The policy sciences* (pp. 3-15). Stanford, CA: Stanford University Press.

Leite, R. W. & Landry Meyer, L. A. (2003). Utilizing assessment in program development and accreditation. *The Journal of Teaching in Marriage and Family, 3*, 267-290.

Lerner, R. M., Sparks, E. E., & McCubbin, L. D. (1999). *Family diversity and family policy: Strengthening families for America's children.* Boston: Kluwer Academic Publishers.

Levine, D. E. (1998). *Remote control childhood? Combating the hazards of media culture.* Washington, DC: National Association for the Education of Young Children.

McAdoo, H. P. (1999). *Family ethnicity: Strengths in diversity* (2nd Ed.). Thousand Oaks, CA: Sage.

Miles, M. & Huberman, M. (1994). *An expanded sourcebook: Qualitative data analysis.* Thousand Oaks, CA: Sage.

Moen, P. & Schorr, A. L. (1987). Families and social policy. In M. B. Sussman & S. K. Steinmetz (Eds.), *Handbook of marriage and the family* (pp. 795-813). New York: Plenum.

Nagel, S. S. (1999). *Teaching public administration and public policy.* Huntington, NY: Nova Science Publishers.

Rotter, J. C. & Casado, M. (1998). Promoting strengths and celebrating culture: Working with Hispanic families. *Family Journal, 6,* 132-141.

Verba, S., Schlozman, K. L., & Brady, H. (1995). *Voice and equality: Civic voluntarism in American politics.* Cambridge, MA: Harvard University Press.

Viramontez Anguiano, R. P. & Harrison, S. M. (2002). Teaching cultural diversity to college students majoring in helping professions: The use of an eco-strength perspective. *College Student Journal, 36,* 152-167.

Zimmerman, S. L. (1995). *Understanding family policy: Theories and applications.* Thousand Oaks, CA: Sage.

# Teaching Family Policy: Advocacy Skills Education

Elaine A. Anderson
Bonnie Braun
Susan K. Walker

**ABSTRACT.** Preparing students to engage in family policy education and advocacy is a challenge and opportunity for departments that teach family studies and family policy courses. Students not only need to know theoretical implications of family policy and how research enhances the theory, but also understand the policy process and how research-based information about family can inform policymaking. These students also need to acquire advocacy skills in order to work effectively in different policy arenas. This article illustrates how university family policy educators can structure curricula to provide students with both knowledge and skills vital to effective participation in family policy formation, analysis and critique. *[Article copies available for a fee from The Haworth Document Delivery Service: 1-800-HAWORTH. E-mail address: <docdelivery@haworthpress.com> Website: <http://www.HaworthPress.com> © 2005 by The Haworth Press, Inc. All rights reserved.]*

**KEYWORDS.** Advocacy skills education, experiential learning, family policy

---

Elaine A. Anderson is Professor, Bonnie Braun is Associate Professor, and Susan K. Walker is Assistant Professor, Department of Family Studies, University of Maryland.

Address correspondence to: Elaine A. Anderson, Professor, Department of Family Studies, University of Maryland, 1204 Marie Mount Hall, College Park, MD 20742 (E-mail: eanders@umd.edu).

## INTRODUCTION

Over the past 20 years, public policy became an integral element in family studies coursework and outreach (Anderson, Zimmerman, & Skinner, 1991; Anderson, 2001). We moved from barely mentioning policy in our classrooms or community-based education programming, to having courses, textbooks (Bogenschneider, 2002; Skinner & Anderson, 1993; Zimmerman, 1995), and special issues of our major journals devoted to the topic of family policy. Furthermore, our professional associations are publishing policy materials for use in classrooms and communities (Anderson, 2004; Anderson, Skinner, & Letiecq, 2004; NCFR, 2000). A family policy course is now required for the National Council on Family Relations' Certified Family Life Educator. Specialists in family policy are hired in academic departments to conduct policy research and teach family policy in our classrooms and through outreach education. Family policy is finally recognized as a central element of the educational curricula of family studies.

Simultaneously the policy arena moved explicitly into the area of family. In the past decade, more policy initiatives at the local, state and federal levels had a family focus. Examples include welfare reform, the Responsible Fatherhood initiatives, and most recently, the emphasis on marriage education and same-sex marriages. Thus two directional shifts occurred: the family field may have successfully "enlightened" policymakers to recognize and consider the role of family when developing policy that emphasizes the well-being of individuals, and policy makers may have successfully drawn family researchers into addressing topics that produce more informed decisions for families.

However, despite increased emphasis on families by both elected officials and government agency personnel, emerging policies often do not have a research component or are not developed in light of the existing research of family policy scientists. Policies that lack a research base result from both the nature of the political process and a failure by family professionals to extend research to policymakers and citizens. Not including family research findings in policy decisions will continue unless students are adequately prepared and encouraged to participate in the policy-making process. This article illustrates how family policy educators can structure the curricula to provide students with knowledge and skills vital to effective participation in family policy formation, analysis and critique.

## DEFINING ADVOCACY

Advocacy has been defined in multiple ways. It can be defined as "lobbying" for a particular piece of legislation or regulation or other public policy. Bogenschneider (2002) suggests advocacy is when one campaigns for an underrepresented group or policy alternative that could enhance family well-being. Others argue the intent of advocacy is to persuade, or as Smith (1991) indicates, advocacy is intended to shape and influence debate by taking a side surrounding a family issue. Professional associations, many organizations and agencies, and units in public education institutions such as Cooperative Extension are either not permitted to lobby or are limited in their lobbying from existing governing laws and internal policies set by their boards of directors. Rather, typically these groups take the role of educator–disseminating research findings to be considered in the decision-making process. Examples of this role are articulated by Nye and McDonald (1979), Bogenschneider (1995b), and the National Council on Family Relations (2004).

Braun and Williams (2002) identify a role for family professionals as advocates for families in policy discussions. They suggest that such advocacy is practiced when professionals urge policy makers to consider family perspectives and utilize research focused on families in their deliberations. Indeed, both family professionals and professional associations frequently present the case for considering family when proposing public policy and when examining the consequences of public policy decisions. Tools such as analytic frameworks are employed to promote family viewpoints. One tool is the "Checklist for Assessing the Impact of Policies and Programs on Families," first published by Ooms and Preister (1988) and later incorporated into "Public Policy Through a Family Lens" (NCFR, 2000).

The increased attention being given to family in social and public policy places family research skills in high demand. As a result, many of our students will face the challenge of applying research findings, and conveying information about family issues in a persuasive and compelling way to policy makers. Students therefore need more than an abstract understanding of the relationship between family and policy. They need solid family research skills, a thorough understanding of the issues and content of a breadth of family life topics, knowledge of the legislative process, and experience in the multiple avenues of advocacy.

In the Department of Family Studies at the University of Maryland, we prepare undergraduate and graduate students to apply theory to family policy issues. We teach them advocacy skills through coursework and applied learning experiences with faculty engaged in public issues education and public policy advocacy so they can effectively communicate their knowledge during the legislative and/or regulatory process. Our students gain first-hand experience in policy arenas through internships in local, state or federal agencies or through a variety of volunteer activities. We strive to develop writing skills, key when presenting and interpreting research findings and building a case for the impact on families of proposed or existing public policy. Our goal is for students to graduate as competent citizens, teachers of family policy and/or professional advocates able to effectively participate in public policy analysis, evaluation and development.

While few other universities or colleges with family studies programs or those that teach family policy courses are located with easy access to both the nation's capital and their own state house, most can find ways to get their students involved in federal policy via travel to Washington, electronic access to policy hearings, briefs, and through direct contact with their Congressional delegation. Family studies departments and departments that teach family policy courses can also create access to their state government and many regional policy-related meetings. Most state legislators have conveniently located regional offices that enable ready access for students with their elected officials and staff. Also, all departments are located in communities where students and faculty can become involved in local public policy as a means of developing advocacy skills. Finally, many family studies departments are fortunate to have faculty with Extension appointments. These educators involve students in community-based projects and public issues education (Patton & Blaine, 2001) that engage citizens in the legislative and/or regulatory policy-making processes across the state.

The following section describes learning experiences for student advocacy skill development. Such skills prepare students to be good public policy educators, enabling them to conduct policy-oriented research and evaluate programs from a policy perspective whether they work in academic, Extension, policy or human service professions. Students in any of these career tracts will recognize the utility of good advocacy skills.

## *ADVOCACY SKILL EDUCATION ACTIVITIES*

What knowledge and skills should students develop to become effective advocates? To effectively engage in public policy activities requires five skills:

- Knowledge of the issue, including the analysis of applicable research findings;
- Understanding of appropriate points of intervention in the public policy development and decision process;
- Familiarity with public policy decision-makers or those who influence them;
- Knowledge about human nature and human interactions; and, finally,
- Persuasive skills for the development and implementation of public policy activities (Anderson & Skinner, 1995).

Each of these policy education aspects related to a university family studies curriculum is outlined below.

## *Gaining Knowledge of Issues*

One way to gain knowledge of public policy issues is to study them in the abstract by reading textbooks or other materials. Another way is for students to learn by engaging in the public policy process as part of their coursework. Pratt (1995) suggests that conducting research, program evaluations, and statutory and policy analyses will advance both the understanding of family policy issues and the processes that produce family policies. Pratt notes that both undergraduate and graduate students would better understand the focus of their policy interests through experiences that allow them to conduct policy research, program evaluations or policy analyses.

In our department, we provide experiences that compliment courses on family policy. We involve undergraduates in research apart from or integrated into their coursework. A required assignment in the research methods class is to conduct a study and to examine the findings in light of public policy. Here graduate students conduct or assist in research projects with a family policy focus. These projects may result from an identified problem in a community, such as homelessness, or may be after a policy, such as welfare reform, is implemented to assess the impact on families.

Graduate students are encouraged to participate with faculty in conducting program evaluations. They get experience communicating with decision makers on the efficacy of the policy behind the program. Not only do students gain advocacy skills, but also local or state social service agencies get external program evaluations of the impact of their programs on families. Courses in program evaluation are also particularly useful. Finally, through conducting statutory and policy analyses our students advance their understanding of family issues within a political context. Some experiences can be gained by voluntarily assisting a group or organization responsible for providing human services. Internships with agencies and associations that conduct policy research also provide enriching experiences. Students learn to analyze findings from program evaluations and ask questions concerning policy impacts on families.

However, we do our students an injustice if we do not provide them with family policy and family law coursework. In addition to sociology and political science departments, public affairs or government and politics departments frequently offer policy courses with opportunities for the analysis of legislation, or the design or implementation of program evaluations. Although the course may not focus specifically on family, course projects may permit the student to concentrate on a family issue. Additionally, there are law courses offered in various disciplines, such as political science and history. Conducting policy analyses in coursework, participating in research where results are interpreted with a policy focus, being involved with a program evaluation to assess the effectiveness of a policy already implemented, and volunteering or undertaking internships with policy analysis groups are all examples of activities where students clearly can become knowledgeable about the issues and policies at hand.

## *Understanding the Legislative and/or Regulatory Decision-Making Process*

The value of understanding the legislative process is shared with a personal example by Bogenschneider (2002). While she was a student intern, she utilized her research and legislative knowledge to produce a background paper on the Special Milk Amendment and its impact on the well-being of low-income children, shared her document with key Democratic and Republican legislators, and helped build a statewide coalition of supportive organizations who advocated for the amendment. The Special Milk Amendment was included in the signed budget bill.

Bogenschneider's understanding of the process by which legislators or other officials make decisions maximized the success of the passage of the policy. Through our departmental public policy education initiatives, we have developed numerous opportunities to engage students in this learning and advocacy process. The sites for these activities include: (1) the Maryland Family Policy Impact Seminar, (2) Cooperative Extension outreach initiatives, (3) internships, and (4) advocacy efforts within our department.

*The Maryland Family Policy Impact Seminar.* Bogenschneider (1995a, 2002) suggests that family professionals can promote a family perspective in state policymaking by informing debates through the presentation of various policy alternatives to family problems. Family Impact Seminars represent one tool that can be used to inform legislators about family issues. To date, twelve states have joined a consortium to develop these seminars. In 2001, the Maryland Family Policy Impact Seminar (MFPIS) was developed.

One of the activities of the MFPIS is to conduct national issues forums (National Issues Forum, 1996) as designed by the Kettering Foundation. These public forums provide Maryland citizens the opportunity to deliberate and discuss matters of family policy, finding common ground and shared direction through their dialogue. Undergraduate and graduate students are involved in organizing and running the forums as well as analyzing the outcomes.

*Cooperative Extension outreach initiatives.* Extension public policy education focuses on applying research to problems and issues and helping citizens and policy makers make informed decisions (Patton & Blaine, 2001). In family departments at land-grant universities with Cooperative Extension faculty appointments, students have the opportunity to join Extension faculty in research projects, program evaluation, and the development of educational materials.

Students involved in Cooperative Extension outreach often gain an understanding of the legislative and/or the regulatory processes. At the University of Maryland, examples include:

1. Development and implementation of a child care policy analysis tool (Walker, Swank, & Oesterriech, 2003) utilized by the public, legislators and their staffs to understand issues in early child care education related to quality care, financing and availability;
2. Participation in leadership development training for a Latino neighborhood that produced an inventory of community needs and assets and then formed a non-profit organization representing immigrant citizens interests in local politics (McClintock-Comeaux & Walker, 2003);
3. Conducting forums and publishing the public's response on the web and through a poster presentation to Congress (Grutzmacher, 2004); and,

4. Attending planning sessions to develop tools to inform state legislators about the impacts of the Medicare Modernization Act of 2003 resulting in the appointment of a subcommittee on prescription drugs (Bohn & Braun, 2004).

Family studies students with an interest in policy, work with Extension faculty to prepare educational material through a review of the research and policy literature, and the creation, testing, and revision of documents. They lead and moderate forums and discussions about salient policy issues and assist in Extension program evaluation. They participate when the fun begins–when programming occurs with the public.

*Internship opportunities.* For over 30 years, the University of Maryland Family Studies Department has required an internship course that serves students well in providing them the opportunity to get "hands on experience." Students become acquainted with the public policy process from the perspective of agencies and organizations outside of the academy. These internships sometimes influence their choice of thesis and dissertation research, selection of career focus, and size of students' network of contacts. There are many settings where students gain policy and advocacy skills (Anderson et al., 2004).

Perhaps the most obvious settings where students may gain exposure to the necessary advocacy skills are in government entities. Students can find a state legislator, who regularly introduces legislation related to children and families, or make contact with the state department of children, youth and families and discuss various internship possibilities. County and city government offices are also entities to consider for internship placements. Each locality and branch of government will provide a different perspective because of the varying public policies that are the domain of federal, state, county, or city government. Private policy research firms offer internships where students can conduct research and develop advocacy skills. Additionally, many private not-for-profit organizations are involved in presenting family perspectives, family research and/or targeted advocacy.

Students can identify these opportunities by monitoring recent legislative hearings regarding their area of interest since organizational representatives frequently testify at hearings or submit written testimony. Students can also determine if special commissions have been established consisting of coalitions of groups or individuals who have common interests and advocacy strategies around specific issues. Examples of these established groups might be women's commissions or commissions for the elderly, a youth involvement commission, or perhaps a child care commission. In many communities, family-focused coalitions of private citizens, professionals, and agencies work together to advocate for policies and programs on behalf of families.

Finally, simply reading the daily newspaper or browsing the Internet can provide information about groups that are advocating for families. Often articles are written in the local newspaper to inform citizens about the various "good will" work conducted by a service organization. Hence, the organization being recognized may be a great source for students looking for an exciting policy/advocacy internship. Helping students to be creative and proactive in looking for their internships should be part of the faculty member's responsibility and a major component of their policy education.

*In-house advocacy.* Sometimes advocacy initiatives arise within the department or university that present an opportunity for students to enhance their understanding of the legislative process and practice their advocacy skills. Our department has a certified program in marriage and family therapy, an area that occasionally becomes the focus of public policy. When the state of Maryland began to consider certification or licensure for marriage and family therapists, our faculty and students got involved. Believing that families are best served by licensed professionals, faculty and students advocated for licensure. Through that initiative our students learned how to develop coalitions with other therapists, write talking points to be utilized when they met with legislators, write succinct letters to legislators to garner their attention on important issues, and develop skills of writing and presenting testimony. In order to track the legislation through the decision-making process, students became experts on how a bill becomes a law and the numerous political and policy actions that could derail such an outcome.

Unlike some policy initiatives that may not have a direct impact on the students, this one did because the marriage and family therapy initiative was very relevant for the future economic livelihood of the students. Such policy work was instrumental in helping students understand the fine nuances of public policy. Students should be encouraged to become involved in their local professional organization and utilize their advocacy skills to address other family policy issues.

## Becoming Familiar with Persons Targeted for Persuasion

The more contact our students have with legislators and decision makers, the greater the opportunities to learn about these persons, their interests, and legislative and/or regulatory processes. When students review a legislator's voting record and position on issues, they gain insight into what policy areas the lawmaker might support. In general, the greater the exposure to decision makers and their staffs over time, the more likely one can become knowledgeable about the dynamics that influence policymakers. There are various settings that will allow students to become more familiar with persons who might be targeted for persuasion.

*Government targets for persuasion.* Perhaps the most obvious avenues for students to familiarize themselves with decision makers is by attending committee hearings and caucuses where questions are raised by legislators in response to testimony. Other situations that expose students to the values and positions of a legislator are meeting with legislative staff to discuss a policy issue the legislator is considering, or participating with legislators in small group tours of human service agencies or related businesses addressing family matters.

Students can serve as aides to faculty who are members of specially appointed legislative commissions. Students often attend commission meetings and assist in preparing materials for discussion. Commission work entails the development of analytic documents and fact sheets utilizing public data backed by scientific research. Students assist faculty by preparing these fact sheets, attending public hearings when the documents are presented, and by tracking the outcomes of policy decisions resulting from their work. Through this activity students continue to enhance their understanding of the legislative process and become more exposed to legislators and their aides while working in another legislative context.

*Non-governmental targets for persuasion.* We should also realize that students could become exposed to policy change agents and their persuasive techniques through settings other than the legislature. Our students are encouraged, and frequently supported financially, to participate in the public policy work of professional associations. Examples of these activities include serving on a national public policy committee, attending policy sessions at professional conferences, and meeting with legislative staff to discuss the policy issues of concern to the association membership and to offer assistance in providing staff with data that may help to better inform policy development and decision making. It is important to inform students about the benefits that such actions could bring for them. These policy engagement opportunities not only allow students to observe professionals working on policy issues, but also enable them further to make contributions through their own experiences while interacting with elected and appointed representatives. Not only do the students benefit, but the professional associations' ability to respond to policy issues also is enhanced through greater member advocacy expertise.

## *Understanding Human Nature and Styles of Interaction*

If politics is the art of the possible, then effectively influencing policy requires understanding how people are influenced. Persuasion succeeds when grounded in values, beliefs and behaviors that influence decisions. Family studies students are well versed in different styles of human interaction and have a keen interest in understanding the dynamics of human and family interaction. For example, those who work in social service agencies or human relations departments recognize the necessity of understanding the various ways that humans interact and communicate with each other and the implications of these actions. Consequently, students can take numerous classes that enhance their abilities to interact and work with others. Communication courses can help develop the skill to advocate, or the ability to convey research findings with policy implications, by teaching good listening, reflective, writing and speaking skills.

At the undergraduate level the course may have various titles including words such as 'helping skills' and 'communication.' Course content should focus on active listening skills as well as verbal and non-verbal response skills. Many family studies departments offer these classes because they are a required component of the CFLE accrediting program (Bredehoft & Cassidy, 1995). Additionally, if a department does not offer such a class, Communications, Counseling, Psychology and Social Work departments are examples of disciplines that may offer such classes under the context of their outreach initiatives. However, knowing about human nature and effectively working with people requires skills gained only through experience. Students must seek opportunities to practice those communication skills and to observe human nature at work in public policy settings. Some students who work with the Maryland Family Policy Impact Seminar enhance their written communication skills through development of the website utilized by citizens and policy makers. Because material on the website is regularly updated, students are challenged to remain familiar with changing family policy issues, family policy resources, family research, and advocacy organizations. Students learn how to write policy briefs based on current departmental research with possible policy implications. Graduate students write policy briefs subsequent to the completion of their thesis or dissertation or through involvement with other departmental research projects. They also create or assist in the development of various family policy impact analysis tools. Therefore, addressing multiple family problems by writing material for the policy website has further enhanced the students' communication skills.

## Gaining Skills in the Techniques of Persuasion

Finally, advocacy skills include the ability to persuade. Perhaps the best example of how our undergraduate and graduate students have enhanced their persuasive skills is the legal debate format they learn in their family law classes. Students learn not only how to clearly identify the merits of a legal case, but they also are required to debate one side of a legal position. To further challenge students' persuasive skills, they often are given the side of a position that they personally do not support and must argue for that perspective regardless of their values and views. This Socratic debate strategy prepares students to be able to collect and analyze information, assess the values present, and argue one perspective of an issue that may have multiple positions.

To gain debate experience, students may seek classes in other departments such as political science, government and politics, sociology and criminal justice. Additionally, many universities offer debate classes or opportunities to join debate teams that can also provide students with valuable persuasive advocacy skills. In our department, a number of students have sharpened their debating skills by joining the university mock trial team. Faculty could also incorporate debate into their class assignments.

Persuasive skills can also be developed through student-designed mass media products created as a class project, or as a volunteer effort to support an advocacy organization. For example, public service announcements (PSAs) are short, carefully timed audio or audio-video pieces delivered to locally broadcast mass media outlets. Condensing a complex issue into a 30-second spot can help students learn how to create talking points, useful in brief meetings with legislators. Students may also want to develop web pages that convey information and a persuasive message about a family policy issue. The use of posters to present information, a frequent format at professional meetings, is another tool that can be used in the communication process.

In 2004, some of our graduate students chose to investigate publicly available family policy positions of the two major presidential candidates. Their resulting "Family Issues Voting Guide" was posted on the departmental Maryland Family Policy Impact Seminar website (University of Maryland Council on Family Relations and Maryland Family Policy Impact Seminar, 2004) and promoted on the homepage of the University of Maryland website. Two family-focused professional associations also promoted the guide. This outreach activity, prepared as part of a family policy graduate class, necessitated students to present two perspectives on each issue. This activity further built the students' communication skills and their ability to present a clear position.

The creation of position statements or policy briefs that build a case for public policy related to specific family issues also teaches persuasion skills. The briefs must concisely convey research findings in language used by the people for whom the brief is written. The policy briefs that our students develop are one method of communicating a case. Another is to present a case orally, such as in testimony, or via op-ed pieces for newspapers. Finally, students learn persuasion when they participate in the issues forums mentioned earlier. The forums are structured to engage participants in the examination of a variety of policy and programmatic approaches and to clarify their views about the tensions among the approaches. Students have built both organizational and persuasive skills as moderators for these forums.

## CONCLUSION

In this article, we presented our case for family policy educators to teach family studies students advocacy skills to be utilized in different policy arenas. We suggested that by obtaining certain knowledge and skills students could become effective advocates for families in the public policy process. We shared approaches undertaken in our department to educate students through coursework, faculty project initiatives and direct experience that engage citizens in public policy with a focus on families (see Table 1).

A next step for our department is to assess the effectiveness of these approaches. We currently rely on comments from students, policy makers, supervisors of internships, and faculty to determine the extent to which the students are learning vital advocacy skills. Our department, and other departments or programs, would benefit by conducting a systematic examination of the degree to which our methods of teaching family policy advocacy actually produce skilled practitioners who effectively participate in the public policy arena. Findings from the

TABLE 1. Strategies for Teaching Advocacy Skills

| Skill | Strategies to Involve Students |
|---|---|
| Gain knowledge of issues | Issue research in class projects, faculty research<br>Evaluate programs provided from policy action<br>Policy analysis in coursework, internships, outreach |
| Understand the decision-making process | Presentation of family policy alternatives to legislators (e.g., Family Impact Seminar)<br>Participation in public issue forum administration<br>Prepare materials, assist with administration of Cooperative Extension/outreach initiatives for community decision-making and advocacy<br>Internships with government agencies/offices, non-profits, policy research firms, coalitions<br>In-house advocacy for department issues (e.g., licensure advocacy) |
| Become familiar with persons involved with the issue | Internships (see above)<br>Attend hearings<br>Aid faculty with work on commissions<br>Aid professional associations with advocacy efforts |
| Gain knowledge about human nature and interactions | Build on students' interest in human interpersonal dynamics natural to those in the family studies profession<br>Additional coursework in human relations, communication, psychology<br>Development of educational tools, policy briefs, and Websites on issues and policies |
| Gain persuasion skills | Debate experience and skill development through course projects/activities (e.g., Mock Trial, hearings)<br>Development of persuasive public education materials (e.g., Public Service Announcements, Web pages, posters)<br>Develop position statements on public issues of interest (e.g., election materials)<br>Participation in issue forums (see above) |

evaluation would be useful for continual program improvement in departments where family policy is included in the curriculum. Findings would also be helpful for those departments that want to add advocacy experiences to their program and would add credence to our case that departments can, and should prepare students to effectively enter the public advocacy arena.

The intent of this article was to challenge family policy educators to engage their students in activities that will develop their advocacy skills, to recognize the important role that advocacy plays in the knowledge base of our family policy students, and to help those teaching family policy to incorporate advocacy information and skill training into their curricula. We were motivated by the belief that if we neglect this important policy education task, then our students will not have the knowledge and skills they need to engage in the important public work that makes a democracy strong. By preparing students through combined classroom and real world learning experiences, we should increase the likelihood that the needs and assets of families will be included in family public policies. Therefore, we ask, if college and university family departments don't teach our undergraduate and graduate students family policy advocacy skills, who will?

## REFERENCES

Anderson, C. (Ed.). (2004). *Family and community policy: Strategies for civic engagement*. Washington, DC: American Association of Family Consumer Sciences.

Anderson, E. A. (2001, November). Family policy education: Course development strategies and resources from a federal perspective. Distinguished scholars roundtable presentation at the meeting of the National Council on Family Relations, Rochester, N.Y.

Anderson, E. A. & Skinner, D. A. (1995). The components of family policy education. *Journal of Family and Economic Issues, 16*, 65-77.

Anderson, E. A., Skinner, D. A., & Letiecq, B. L. (Eds.). (2004). *Teaching family policy: A handbook of course syllabi, teaching strategies and resources*. Minneapolis, MN: National Council on Family Relations.

Anderson, E. A., Zimmerman, S., & Skinner, D.A. (1991, November). Teaching a course on family policy. Paper presented at the meeting of the National Council on Family Relations, Denver, CO.

Bredehoft, D. & Cassidy, D. (Eds). (1995). *College and university curriculum guidelines in family life education curriculum*. Minnesota: National Council on Family Relations. Retrieved on March 12, 2005 from http://www.ncfr.org/pdf/FLE_Substance_Areas.pdf

Bogenschneider, K. (1995a, October). Promoting a family perspective in policy making with state family impact seminars. Paper presented at Expert Meeting, Leuven, Belgium.

Bogenschneider, K. (1995b). Roles for professionals in building family policy: A case study of state family impact seminars. *Family Relations, 44*, 5-12.

Bogenschneider, K. (2002). *Family policy matters: How policymaking affects families and what professionals can do*. Mahwah, NJ: Lawrence Erlbaum Associates.

Bohn, J. & Braun, B. (2004). *Prescription drug policy analysis tool*. Retrieved on March 17, 2005 from: http://www.hhp.umd.edu/FMST/fis/current.html

Braun, B. & Williams, S. (2002). We the people: Renewing commitment to civic engagement. *Journal of Family and Consumer Sciences, 94*, 8-16.

Grutzmacher, S. (2004). *Examining health care: What's the public's prescription?* Retrieved on March 17, 2005 from http://www.hhp.umd.edu/FMST/fis/ mdresources.html

McClintock-Comeaux, M. & Walker, S. (2003). *Leadership community development program in the Langley Park community: Liderazgo. Final evaluation report*. College Park, MD: University of Maryland, Maryland Cooperative Extension.

National Council on Family Relations. (2000). *Public policy through a family lens: Sustaining families in the 21st century.* Minneapolis, MN: Author.

National Council on Family Relations. (2004). *Family science: Professional development and career opportunities.* Minneapolis, MN: Author.

National Issues Forum Institute. (1996). *The troubled American family: Which way out of the storm?* Washington, DC: Author.

Nye, F. I. & McDonald, G. W. (1979). Family policy research: Emergent models and some theoretical issues. *Journal of Marriage and the Family, 41,* 473-485.

Ooms, T. & Preister, S. (Eds.). (1988). *A strategy for strengthening families: Using family criteria in policymaking and program evaluation.* Washington, DC: Family Impact Seminar.

Patton, D. B. & Blaine, T. W. (2001). Public issues education: Exploring Extension's role. *Journal of Extension, 39.* Retrieved on March 29, 2004 from www.joe.org/joe/2001august/a2.html.

Pratt, C. (1995). Family professionals and family policy: Strategies for influence. *Family Relations, 44,* 56-62.

Skinner, D. A. & Anderson, E. A. (Eds.). (1993). *Teaching family policy: A handbook of course syllabi, teaching strategies and resources.* Minneapolis, MN: National Council on Family Relations.

Smith, J.A. (1991). *The idea brokers: Think tanks and the rise of the new policy elite.* New York: The Free Press.

University of Maryland Council on Family Relations and Maryland Family Policy Impact Seminar. (2004). *An election guide.* Retrieved on March 22, 2005 from http://www.hhp.umd.edu/FMST/fis/_docs/Family_Election_Guide.pdf

Walker, S., Swank, C., & Oesterreich, L. (2003). *Early care and education programs and policies: A checklist.* (Extension Cares Initiative, CSREES). Washington DC: USDA.

Zimmerman, S. (1995). *Understanding family policy: Theoretical approaches.* Newbury Park, CA: Sage.

# Involving Marginalized Families in Shaping Policies: Roles for Cooperative Extension

Kimberly Greder
Jeanne Warning

**ABSTRACT.** Family involvement in the policy-making process is critical to ensuring that policies are designed to effectively address family needs. This manuscript identifies critical roles for cooperative extension and other educators in involving families in shaping policies. Two educational tools, *Sharing a Family's Story* and the *ROWEL Poverty Simulation*, that assist in bringing a family perspective to policy making are described. *[Article copies available for a fee from The Haworth Document Delivery Service: 1-800-HAWORTH. E-mail address: <docdelivery@haworthpress.com> Website: <http://www.HaworthPress.com> © 2005 by The Haworth Press, Inc. All rights reserved.]*

**KEYWORDS.** Capacity building, cooperative extension, family issues, family policy, marginalized families

---

Kimberly Greder is Assistant Professor, Human Development & Family Studies and Family Life Extension State Specialist, and Jeanne Warning is Assistant Director to Families, Iowa State University.

Address correspondence to: Kimberly Greder, PhD, CFLE, CFCS, Assistant Professor, Human Development & Family Studies and Family Life Extension State Specialist, 56 LeBaron Hall, Iowa State University, Ames, IA 50011-1120 (E-mail: kgreder@iastate.edu).

## INTRODUCTION

Cooperative Extension educators have an important role to play in helping the public understand critical issues facing families and how people, individually and collectively, can influence policy. The purpose of this article is to describe two educational tools that can be used to assist marginalized families, those who do not have equal access to power and are often left out of the policy-making process, in influencing programs and policies.

If policies and programs are developed with the intent of supporting families, then it is essential that families be involved as an equal voice in the formulation of the very policies and programs that directly affect their lives. Therefore, it is critical that families be viewed not just as consumers, but as politically engaged citizens (Doherty, 2000). "A policy focus on government services that does not include a strong component of partnership with families ultimately can undermine families and democracy itself" (Doherty, 2000, p. 321). Innovative solutions often rest on a willingness to negotiate, share power, and explore collaborative action (National Public Policy Education Committee, 2002). Therefore, strengthening families' capacity to tell their stories can help them become more involved in the decision-making process (Greder et al., 2004).

While working with all families is important, we focus our attention on families who do not have equal access to power, and are not often heard during the policy-making process. Such families are often marginalized by poverty, disability, and other special challenges, including undocumented residence status in the United States. They are at greater risk for poor child outcomes than families who do not face these special challenges. For example, families who experience poverty are at greater risk for infant mortality, undernourishment, child abuse and neglect, poor health, substance abuse, teenage pregnancy, violence, crime, and academic underachievement (Kids Count, 2004; Mayer, 1997).

In the long term, children marginalized by poverty are at risk for not becoming responsible family members or productive citizens. Health care, remedial education, foster care, incarceration, and welfare costs continue to rise as the needs of these children increase (Children, Youth and Families At Risk Program, 2005). The Cooperative Extension System, as a component of the Land-Grant University system, is directly involved with families throughout the U.S. and particularly with low-income families. Understanding the values, priorities, needs, dreams, and experiences of such families will help service providers and policy makers design more effective programs and policies (Greder, 2003a).

Involving marginalized families in the program and policy decision-making process may not be easy because their personal challenges may be so great that they have little time, energy, or resources to participate in larger community programs. They are not politically organized and are often disconnected from community political systems and power structures (McLeroy, Bibeau, Steckler, & Glanz, 1988). However, it is essential that families become involved in identifying problems, organizing for action, and seeking solutions (Doherty, 2000).

For many families, financial support may be needed to help off-set the costs of child care, transportation, or absenteeism from work due to community organizing and other types of advocacy activities (Greder et al., 2004). Family professionals need to develop creative strategies to address the above barriers in order for families to participate in the program and policy decision-making process. Two educational tools designed to assist families in learning how to inform policy at various levels are discussed below.

## TWO EDUCATIONAL TOOLS FOR INFORMING POLICY AND BUILDING CAPACITY

*Sharing a Family's Story* and the *ROWEL Poverty Simulation* are examples of educational efforts that directly involve families. These programs utilize different teaching techniques and provide opportunities for families to share their experiences, values and goals with policy makers and program staff.

### Sharing a Family's Story

The resource professionals can use to help families share their stories is *Sharing a Family's Story*, a 15-minute videotape and lesson guide. This resource provides examples of family stories and describes methods for helping families develop and share their stories as well as help professionals and others connect intellectually and emotionally with the life experiences of families who face non-normative challenges (Greder, 2003a). These may include divorce, teenage parenthood, poverty, or raising a child with a disability. This intellectual and emotional connection helps professionals to better understand the impact of social service programs and policies on the daily lives of families and their children.

The videotape communicates the stories of three families of diverse backgrounds who face non-normative family challenges. Sonya, a rural Caucasian mother in her 30s, has three young children who have autism. She shares what is important to her and her husband in raising their children, describes special services her family needs, and describes attitudes and actions of service providers and others in the community who are either effective or ineffective in addressing her family's problems.

Marlen, a recent immigrant from Guatemala, is learning to speak English and raise her three young children in a very rural area of the United States. She explains why she and her husband moved from Guatemala, the type of employment opportunities they have had, and describes the challenges they experience in raising their children in the U.S.

Sean, an African American father in his 20s, has joint custody of his son with his former spouse and is striving to eliminate the need for public assistance. Sean describes how public assistance and agency professionals have helped his family meet their needs, and identifies the barriers his family has encountered in accessing the support they need to be self-sufficient (Greder, 2003b).

*Sharing a Family's Story* is designed to assist human service professionals as they work with families and become familiar with their values, goals, priorities, and aspirations. By viewing families as partners instead of faceless recipients of services, human service professionals gather crucial information that helps to improve programs and inform policies. This process not only helps families to survive, but moves them closer to a higher quality of life over the long haul.

Parents share their stories individually and through panel presentations at professional meetings and conferences, and in-service training sessions. Other venues include college/university classrooms, legislative hearings, or meetings with school teachers, administrators and students. Through this process parents are better able to understand their past in relation to an imagined future for themselves and their children, and develop relationships with professionals and others. They report that through sharing their experiences they broaden their experiences, adapt better to new situations, and strive to create change. Through their stories they are able to: (1) turn grief and anger into constructive energy by talking publicly; (2) reinforce their values that guide their commitment to themselves and their children; (3) influence public opinion by illustrating how policies affect families; (4) help themselves and others feel less alone as they strive for change; and (5) convey to legislators and other policymakers the importance of early intervention programs (Gabbard, 1998). An example of how family stories impact professionals is illustrated by the following quote from a preschool director:

> ... the connection and empathy I feel with others–parents and professionals alike–is so powerful when I hear stories that connect somehow with my own. I get tired sometimes of hearing broad statements about how important collaboration is in thinking about family-centered services and programs. What really makes a difference for me is when I hear stories about what happened today at the center . . . what kind of difference we made in the lives of the families we serve. (Gabbard, 1998, p. 4)

Through sharing their stories with key decision makers, parents can facilitate policy makers' understanding of the realities and complexities of their family situations, and the types of policies needed to help them fulfill their basic family functions. A quote from one parent illustrates this point:

> There is so much misinformation in our state about inclusion and natural environments. Recently, I testified at our local school committee meeting and told them how my son was part of his local little league team, even though he uses a wheelchair. A few of the committee people came up later to thank me for showing them some real examples of what we mean by including everyone. (Gabbard, 1998, p. 5)

After hearing parents with limited resources describe how they meet their family food needs on a daily basis, food pantry coordinators concluded that their practices were based on outdated information and not on the needs of families. A quote by a single middle-age Caucasian mother of three young boys illustrates this point: "I know places where I can get free bakery items, free donations. I use those as part of our total family meals" (Greder, 2000, p. 155). Additionally, when a parent shares his/her family story, other parents who face similar circumstances are reminded that they are not alone (Gabbard, 1998), as illustrated in this quote by a 20 year old African American single father:

> I'm coping with it, especially when I was on welfare assistance, by surrounding myself with people who are willing to see me, or who

are willing to help me in that role to self-sufficiency. Being in a local community group of consumers and also those on public assistance who share their stories and build relationships is helpful because one of the biggest barriers that families on welfare face is isolation. (Greder, 2003b)

Family stories vary in focus and in length (thirty seconds to an hour or more). Some parents share what living with their special challenge is like on a daily basis and identify a variety of coping strategies. Other parents talk about policies or services that help them acquire needed services and often discuss particular aspects of policies that create difficulties for them. Inviting parents to share their experiences and perspectives with current and future family professionals will help sensitize human service providers to the strengths and needs of families (McBride, Sharp, Haines, & Whitehead, 1995). Parents are uniquely qualified to provide insights, perspectives, and experiences that may not be otherwise available to professionals and students (Winton & DiVenere, 1995).

An example of where parents have shared their family stories with professionals is during parent panel presentations, a component of *Partnering with Parents*, a training series for family professionals offered by Iowa State University Extension. The primary goals of the parent panels are to (1) increase awareness of the values, needs, and priorities of families facing specific special challenges; (2) identify family strengths; (3) identify family coping strategies; and (4) identify ways service providers can best support families (Greder et al., 2002). During *Partnering with Parents*, three to, four parents who face special challenges (e.g., divorce, drug addiction, parenting a child with a disability, teenage parenting) serve on a parent panel that lasts anywhere from an hour to 90 minutes during the training. Parents respond to a variety of questions from professionals who are attending the training.

- What is the most important value you want to instill in your child(ren)?
- How has the special challenge you face influenced how you parent your child(ren)?
- How has the special challenge you face as a family changed you? Your family?
- Share with us the type of information and support you and your family want and need from service providers in your community. Are there particular people that have been helpful to you and your

family? If so, who are they and how have they been helpful? What is it about them that has made you feel comfortable and trust them?
- Describe what didn't go well in the ways services were delivered and what you wished had happened. Be specific.

Parents are also invited to join the professionals in small group discussions and other learning activities for the remainder of the day to help professionals to gather information in a more personal format. *Partnering with Parents* facilitators meet with parents in advance to prepare them for the panel presentation. Facilitators share background information about the professionals who participate in the training (e.g., job titles), the format of the panel presentation, and sample questions to address in their presentations (e.g., a brief description of their family structure, the unique challenge they face) (Greder et al., 2002; Greder et al., 2004).

Family professionals who participated in *Partnering with Parents* report that the parent panels provided them opportunities to ask questions that they may not otherwise feel comfortable asking the families they serve. Family professionals report that hearing from parents directly, and then debriefing them as a group, helped them to better identify family strengths, understand the importance of applying family-centered principles to their work with families, and understand more fully the complexities of family life (Greder, 2004).

Parents believe that family professionals in general have some inaccurate information about marginalized families, which affects how they interact with them, as illustrated in the following quotes by two mothers in their 30s (Greder et al., 2004). A 32 year old Mexican immigrant mother of two young children stated:

> Yes. It is good they (agency staff) know because sometimes they only think we are the way it is in the TV ... Sometimes we don't have everything in Mexico that we have here, but we have similar things ... it would be really interesting to share that. (Greder et al., 2004, p. 102)

A Caucasian mother, 36 years old, who recently returned home to her two young children and teenage daughter from a drug rehabilitation program declared:

> I think it does provide some firsthand training and experience to these agencies. You know, you can only learn so much in a book. After that ... every individual is different .... I think that (training)

should happen . . . because these parents are giving these students some insight, you know, what it is really like. (Greder et al., 2004, p. 102)

Factors that prevented parents from participating on panels included a lack of time, limited or no access to child care during presentations, language barriers for immigrants in particular, and loss of income due to absences from work in order to participate in panels (Greder et al., 2004). A Mexican father of three young children stated that although it is important to share his perspectives with professionals, it can be intimidating sometimes.

> Sharing our experiences and perspectives could be helpful. . . . It's like moving to another world (moving to the U. S.) and we are doing a different thing. . . . They gonna say we didn't tell you to come here, you came because you wanted to and you want to change it. . . . Sometimes we don't get involved because we think they (agency staff) are going to make fun of us or how we live in Mexico. They think nobody wants to go there and there is no good there. But, there is good in Mexico and it is a good idea to share that (with agency staff). (Greder et al., 2004, p. 102)

Parents can also be invited to university classrooms to share their family stories with undergraduate and graduate students who are preparing to become family professionals. In 2002, two Iowa State University undergraduate students reported on the value of listening to the family stories that parents shared in their child development class. The course they participated in focused on the needs of families who had children who were at risk for developmental delays (Greder et al., 2004). One university student in her early 20s emphasized that hearing directly from parents made the content of the course seem more applicable.

> Through the stories parents shared about their lives, I have learned a great deal more than by reading a book. It put a face and emotions on the "families" we are always talking about in our class activities. It has helped me see what kind of lives parents may be living when all I otherwise would have thought about was the child. Getting to actually hear from parents helps me to better understand the purpose of being family-centered and how important it is. (Greder et al., 2004, p. 107)

Another student emphasized that listening to parents influenced how she will interact with families in the future.

> I have been so impacted by the personal stories of the families that I will never look at working with a child in the same way. I no longer have such a narrow perspective that focuses only on the child. That child is now a part of something larger, involving the whole family and the needs of so many other people. I hope that I will continue to grow in my understanding of the concept of supporting the whole family. (Greder et al., 2004, p. 107)

A parent of two children with learning and emotional disabilities revealed the following thoughts after sharing her story with students in a course.

> It is empowering. Gets me time to think about what should be happening in our community and in our own situation. I learn what is being recommended so I could try and do this for my family. It was a good thing because it gave me time to sit back and think about where we were before, where we are now and how far we have come.... The best part was the fact they wanted to know my viewpoint. I felt like what a parent has to say does matter. That doesn't happen in very many situations. (Greder et al., 2004, p. 107)

Involving parents in sharing their family stories does make an impact on the attitudes and behaviors of students training to be professionals, as well as on professionals who are actively working with families. Another educational tool that helps increase professionals' understanding of the perspectives and experiences of marginalized families is the ROWEL poverty simulation.

## *ROWEL Poverty Simulation*

One teaching technique that promotes experiential learning is the ROWEL poverty simulation, a well-designed activity in which learners live through a "real-life" situation. Participants assume an assigned role and experience the consequences of their decisions as they respond to particular situations (Greder, 1992). Created by the Reform Organization of Welfare (ROWEL) Education Association of Missouri, the ROWEL poverty simulation (www.extension.iastate.edu/cyfar/simulation) is aimed at professionals and other community members from middle to high-income backgrounds who have never experienced poverty and lack an understanding of the issues that poor families encounter daily (Shirer, Klemme, & Broshar, 1998).

The simulation takes approximately 2.5 to 3 hours to complete and includes an introduction and preparation period, the simulation itself, and a debriefing session. Experience in conducting the simulation in Iowa has led to the conclusion that the ideal group size for effectively implementing it is 30-80 participants (Shirer et al., 1998). Family profiles that are assumed by the participants include newly unemployed parents, single parents with small children applying for welfare benefits and food stamps, undocumented residents who have limited incomes, and elderly persons who receive Social Security and Medicaid benefits. Each "family" receives a packet of information that describes their family structure, financial resources, expenses (e.g., medical bills, rent) and needs (e.g., medical care, child care). There are four 15-minute periods representing one week each. During each week families attempt to meet their food, housing, medical and other needs through interacting with other family members, and various community agencies and organizations. Volunteer "staffers" (people who have experienced poverty) play the roles of community service providers (e.g., food stamp clerk, WIC clerk, food pantry worker, elementary school teacher, bank loan officer, landlord, etc.) and are located at tables around the perimeter of the room.

Following the one-hour simulation, participants and staffers meet in small groups to listen to participants' experiences and insights that occurred during the simulation. One participant from each small group then shares highlights from their group's discussion with the larger group. After listening to participants, staffers share with the larger group their observations of the behaviors and attitudes displayed by participants during the simulation. The staffers also comment on whether or not the behaviors and attitudes demonstrated are consistent with those of families who experience poverty. The staffers often reveal personal stories that provide insight into the decision-making process they used to meet their basic living needs. The dialogue that occurs during this debriefing period helps to increase participants' understanding of specific attitudes and behaviors of service providers, as well as policies that either help or hinder people's ability to meet their family's basic living needs. This exchange of experiences and perspectives provides an opportunity to enhance the quality of public decisions, thus strengthening policies affecting families (National Public Policy Education Committee, 2002).

Iowa State University Extension began conducting ROWEL poverty simulations in Iowa during 1995 to sensitize communities to the plight of poor families, and to initiate program and policy changes that are more supportive of poor families. Anecdotal reports from participants who were involved in the simulation revealed that the activity was a powerful and emotional experience (Shirer et al., 1998). The ISU Extension project staff perceived there was a need to determine more specific individual and community outcomes resulting from people's participation in the simulation. As a result, a program evaluation was designed and completed for the twenty simulations held during 1996 and 1997.

Qualitative and quantitative methods were used to collect data for the program evaluation. These included: (1) a written survey distributed to participants immediately following the simulation; (2) focus group interviews; and (3) a written survey mailed to individuals one year after they participated in the simulation.

On the survey that was distributed immediately following the simulation, participants rated their level of understanding after and before the simulation of issues facing poor families, on a scale of 1 to 5 (1 = no understanding; 5 = almost complete understanding) (see Appendix A). This survey utilized the post-pre method of evaluation which includes a retrospective pretest after an educational intervention as a means of minimizing response-shift bias. A traditional pretest-posttest evaluation was not used because it could result in an inaccurate assessment of the impact of the simulation. Participants may have limited knowledge at the beginning of the simulation that prevents them from accurately assessing their baseline understanding of the issues poor families experience. By the end of the simulation, their new understanding of the issues poor families face may have an impact on their responses on the survey. If a pretest was used at the beginning of the simulation, participants have no way to correct an answer at the end of the simulation if they made an inaccurate assessment of their understanding on the pretest (baseline data) (Rockwell & Kohn, 1989).

The evaluation results from 872 evaluations (participants in 20 simulations) revealed significant positive change in understanding on four of the five statements. Paired T-test analysis of the mean scores of the pre- and post-test responses to the five statements are presented in Table 1. These results show that participation in a poverty simulation significantly ($p < .05$) increased their understanding of the financial pressures and stresses faced by poor families. In addition, participants better understood the positive and negative impacts that providers and other

TABLE 1. Changes in Participants' Attitude and Understanding of Poverty

| Item | Mean Post | Pre | T-test |
|---|---|---|---|
| The financial pressure faced by low-income families in meeting basic needs. | 4.00 | 3.24 | .025** |
| The difficult choices people with low resources need to make each month when stretching limited income. | 4.04 | 3.19 | .012** |
| The difficulties in improving one's situation and becoming self-sufficient on a limited income. | 3.99 | 3.12 | .60* |
| The emotional stresses and frustrations created by having limited resources. | 4.11 | 3.23 | .013** |
| The positive and negative impact of "helpers" on people with limited resources. | 3.91 | 3.11 | .002** |

\*\* significant at .05 alpha
\* not significant at .05 alpha

helpers can have on poor people. However, the simulation did not appear to significantly change participants' understanding of the difficulty people on welfare face in trying to become self-sufficient (Shirer et al., 1998).

The various sources of program evaluation data (i.e., survey distributed immediately after the simulation, focus group transcripts, one-year follow-up survey) revealed that the poverty simulation was a useful tool for educating individuals about the reality of poverty. In addition, the follow-up survey revealed that sensitivity and awareness acquired through the simulation were retained by most participants one year later. Eighty-five percent of the respondents to the follow up survey (n = 42) agreed or strongly agreed that the poverty simulation helped them understand what it is like to live in poverty (Shirer et al., 1998).

The data from the two focus groups (n = 18 people) and the follow-up survey (n = 42) revealed that increased personal awareness and understanding of poverty acquired through the simulation did not automatically translate into changes in programs and policies that affect poor families. Some respondents indicated that they were not in a position to affect these changes. Other respondents stated that current federal rules and regulations restrained them from taking action. While respondents reported little concrete action in changing programs and policies, 50% (n = 21) of the respondents in the follow-up survey indicated specific changes they or their organization were planning to make or had made after the poverty simulation (Shirer et al., 1998). The percentage of respondents who identified each change is presented in Table 2.

One example of an indirect way a local policy was changed as a result of the simulation is described as follows. Three respondents worked with their local school district to modify the required list of elementary school supplies in order to make them more affordable for poor families. The school changed the supply list to include non-name brand supplies (e.g., scissors that are not the "Fisker" brand, generic brand glue and crayons). These respondents also continued to meet with school administrators and teachers to identify processes to more effectively connect poor families with community resources.

The findings from this study revealed that additional activities are needed within a community to change programs and policies. A poverty simulation alone typically does not create change. Community groups that conduct simulations need to continue to build their coalitions, carry out needs assessments, identify resources and strengths in their communities, examine options, and develop specific action plans to influence local programs and policies. The poverty simulation is more likely to affect program and policy changes when conducted by an existing community coalition that has identified community assets and needs and is using the simulation as one of several strategies to reach its goals.

Between 1995 and the spring of 2005, more than 10,000 individuals across the state of Iowa participated in ROWEL poverty simulations (Iowa State University Extension, 2004). Local Extension staff organized simulations in partnership with local community organizations

TABLE 2. Ways to Change Services and Programs

| Service or Program | Percent of yes responses | N (42) |
|---|---|---|
| Increase communication among service agencies | 40.0 | 17 |
| Increase public awareness of available services | 33.0 | 14 |
| Make printed materials available in Spanish | 20.0 | 8 |
| Provides poverty simulation experience for all employees | 18.0 | 8 |
| Involve clients in coalition activities and planning efforts | 15.0 | 6 |
| Hire people who can speak Spanish | 13.0 | 5 |
| Make printed materials easier to read | 10.0 | 4 |
| Provide educational programs to clients about policies and programs | 10.0 | 4 |
| Provide computer networking among agencies | 8.0 | 3 |
| Extend service hours beyond 8:00-5:00 | 8.0 | 3 |
| Offer service in satellite locations | 5.0 | 2 |

and institutions, including community action agencies, faith-based organizations, schools, and public health agencies. State Extension specialists have been asked to organize simulations for selected groups, such as volunteers, high school and college students, school teachers and school administrators, WIC staff, community action agency staff, and others. Several thousand other individuals have participated in the simulation conducted by Extension staff in other states across the nation. The experience influences participants' sensitivity to the plight of the poor and provides families with limited incomes an opportunity to open dialogues with key persons directly involved in shaping policy and implementing changes.

The simulation has been conducted in the traditional classroom setting at several educational levels–middle schools, high schools, colleges and universities. One of the challenges confronting instructors is covering the financial costs of the activity. A middle school teacher who incorporated the simulation in her course was able to secure private financial contributions to cover the costs. A high school instructor, also through private contributions, was able to conduct the simulation during the school day in which one hundred and ten high school students participated. The teacher stated that he believed most adolescents are not aware of what many families have to go through to meet daily needs, including the costs of transportation, utilities and food.

University faculty of an undergraduate sociology course and a graduate counselor education course required students ($n = 162$) to participate in one of two poverty simulations offered in the evenings on campus by Iowa State University Extension. Each student paid a small registration fee to help cover the cost. In the future, these faculty plan to add a poverty simulation participant fee to the course delivery fee. Other possibilities might be to seek grants or departmental funding.

University students in these courses indicated that the most meaningful part of the simulations was hearing the real-life stories of the people who experience poverty and played the role of "staffers" during the simulation. The information and perspectives of the staffers made it clear to the students that stereotypes of poor people are not always accurate. The debriefing period following the simulation was critical to processing the thoughts and feelings of the students regarding their experiences during the exercise.

The students who played the role of children in the simulation reported feeling less involved and consequently believed they learned less than those who played the adult roles (e.g., parents). In order to make the experience more meaningful for all participants, a recommendation from some learners was to have participants switch roles (e.g., from an adult role to a child role and vice versa) halfway through the simulation.

One faculty member reported that several students in her class stated that they will try to listen more carefully to families who experience poverty and not judge their behaviors so quickly. The following quotes (Broshar, 2005) illustrate insights gained by university students through participating in the simulations. "I will never talk to families in the same way I have been . . . I now understand their frustrations." "I didn't realize before, that getting food stamps and welfare was such an ordeal. I guess I always thought they came in the mail." "Before the simulation, I think I looked at people in poverty as being people who made poor choices and managed their money poorly . . . I learned that sometimes the check just doesn't stretch far enough. I learned that it can happen to anyone."

Additional information about the ROWEL poverty simulation can be found at www.extension.iastate.edu/cyfar/simulation.

## *CONCLUSION*

The two educational efforts, *Sharing a Family's Story* and the ROWEL poverty simulation, described in this paper are educational tools that call for professionals to serve as catalysts for families who want to influence the very policies that affect their lives (Doherty, 2000). Both tools assist community members and policy makers in learning about the needs of marginalized families.

Cooperative Extension has a critical role to play in involving families in shaping programs and policies. We might think about Cooperative Extension's contribution at two levels. First, we build the capacity of individuals and families to assist them in meeting their needs. Part of that role is to help families learn to communicate their values, goals, wants, needs, and experiences by encouraging them to share their own personal stories at the local level. As suggested in this paper, we focus on listening to the stories of individuals and families who many times have less access to power and are often left out of the decision-making process. Second, at another level our role is to assist communities by bringing individuals and families together to create change. Extension engages citizens in identifying and addressing needs of children, youth and families in their own neighborhoods and communities.

Future roles for extension staff include assisting other family professionals in helping families share their stories, as illustrated by the publication, *Sharing a Family's Story*, which provides concrete ideas for helping families learn to share their stories (Greder, 2003a). Another potential role for extension professionals in the policy arena is that of serving as a catalyst in bringing families and communities together to apply a community partnership model to an issue of concern. Partnership models involve a community asset approach that emphasizes building community resources and expertise that can be used for addressing problems. In a partnership model families identify the issue they want to focus on and the expertise that exists among them. They determine what information is needed in order for them to develop strategies and implement plans (Gillespie, 2004; Doherty, 2000). The extension professional would function in multiple roles in the partnership model. He/she may begin as a catalyst to bring people together, and then move to the roles of facilitator, educator, and initial report writer to nurture the fact finding and decision-making process of the group (Doherty, 2000). A critical aspect of a partnership model is that it goes beyond the understanding that is gained from research to integrating the information with action in community-directed change programs (Gillespie, 2004). Through tools such as *Sharing a Family's Story* and the ROWEL poverty simulation, extension professionals can assist parents in developing their skills and confidence and encourage them to share their experiences and become connected to others in the community. The "others" may include neighbors, service providers, and individuals who are directly involved in designing services and making policies. These tools can be a starting point that eventually leads to involving marginalized families in a project using the community partnership model.

These processes are not without challenges. Extension staff must be clear about their role as educators versus advocates. In a very general sense we are indeed advocates, advocates for effective policies for families. However, as educators, and because we are supported by public revenues, we must be open to encouraging a wide variety of perspectives, and be able and willing to identify policy options in the decision making process.

Integral to this are other challenges. We must recognize that values underlie policy. As individuals, our past experiences, values and personal biases influence how we perceive situations and how we make decisions. We need to acknowledge this and yet ensure that all perspectives are heard and considered in the process. Families can offer us new ways of understanding how policies directly and indirectly affect their lives and how programs should be changed to better meet the needs of families. To achieve this, we must recognize that families are the ultimate source of the information that we call research data (Doherty, 2000). We must also believe in the competence of the families to provide us important policy information. Then, families can be empowered to continue their quest for a better way of life. The tools presented in this paper provide opportunities to directly involve families in educating professionals and policy makers about the values, goals, strengths, and needs of marginalized families and how policies and programs can be designed to effectively meet family needs.

## REFERENCES

Broshar, D. (March, 2005). ROWEL Poverty Simulation Participant Interview, Ames, IA.
Children, Youth and Families At Risk Program (CYFAR) (n.d.). Retrieved April 11, 2005, from http://www.csrees.usda.gov/nea/family/cyfar/cyf-philo.pdf
Doherty, W. J. (2000). Family science and family citizenship: Toward a model of community partnership with families. *Family Relations, 49,* 319-325.
Gabbard, G. (1998, Spring). Family experiences: Ways to lead change through telling your story. *Early Childhood Bulletin, Federation for Children with Special Needs.* Boston, MA.
Gillespie, A. (2004, March). Community plant food project: Linking families and community systems. Retrieved April 11, 2005, from www.cardi.cornell.edu/health_and_safety/food/000284.php
Greder, K. (2000). *A grounded theory: Coping with low income to meet family food and nutrition needs.* Unpublished doctoral dissertation. Iowa State University.
Greder, K., Oesterreich, L., Anderson, P., Kaufman, M. B., Santiago, A., Hegland, S., & McDonnell, S. (2002). Partnering with parents: Walking the journey together. Iowa State University Extension Publication SP 175.
Greder, K. (2003a). Sharing a family's story: A tool for family advocacy. Iowa State University Extension Publication SP 215, Ames, IA. Retrieved May 2004, from www.extension.iastate.edu/Publications/SP215.pdf
Greder, K. (2003b). Sharing a family's story. Video. Iowa State University Extension.
Greder, K. (2004, June). Partnering with parents: Strengthening parenting education as a profession. *NCFR Report.*
Greder, K., Brotherson, M. J., & Garasky, S. (2004). Listening to the voices of marginalized families. In Anderson, C.L. (Ed.), *Family and community policy: Strategies for civic engagement* (pp. 95-116). Alexandria, VA: American Association of Family and Consumer Sciences.
Greder, M. E. (1992). *Designing and evaluating games and simulations: A process approach.* Longa, London, UK: Kogan Page Publishing.
Iowa State University Extension (2004). The ROWEL Poverty Simulation. Retrieved May, 2004, from www.extension.iastate.edu/cyfar/welreforminfo/sim/past.html
Kids Count Data Book (2004). Washington, DC: Produced for the Annie E. Casey Foundation by Population Reference Bureau, 2004. Retrieved April 11, 2005, from www.aecf.org/kidscount/databook/summary/summary11.htm

Mayer, S. E. (1997). *What money can't buy: Family income and children's life chances.* Cambridge, MA: Harvard University Press.

McBride, S. L., Sharp, L., Hains, A. H., & Whitehead, A. (1995). Parents as co-instructors in preservice training: A pathway to family-centered practice. *Journal of Early Intervention, 19,* 377-389.

McLeroy, K. R., Bibeau, D., Steckler, A., & Glanz, K. (1988). An ecological perspective on health promotion programs. *Health Education Quarterly, 15,* 351-377.

National Public Policy Education Committee (NPPEC), Cooperative Extension, Public Issues Education Competencies Task Force (2002). Public Issues Education: Increasing Competence, Enabling Communities. Retrieved April 11, 2005, from www.publicissueseducation.net/links/pie_black.pdf

Rockwell, S.K. & Kohn H. (1989). Post-then-pre evaluation. *Journal of Extension, 27* (2). Retrieved May 12, 2005, from http://www.joe.org/joe/1989summer/a5.html

Shirer, K., Klemme, D., & Broshar, D. (1998). The Iowa Experience with the ROWEL Poverty Simulation. Iowa State University Extension. Retrieved May 2004, from http://www.extension.iastate.edu/cyfar/welreforminfo/sim/index.html

Winton, P. J. & DiVenere, N. (1995). Family-professional partnerships in early intervention personnel preparation: Guidelines and strategies. *Topics in Early Childhood Special Education, 15,* 296-313.

## APPENDIX A
Written survey questions addressing participants' understanding of poverty.

Directions: Read each of the statements and rank yourself at the present time. Next, think back to your understanding about each statement before you participated in the poverty simulation. Circle the appropriate number using the following key:

1 = no understanding
2 = little understanding
3 = moderate understanding
4 = quite a bit of understanding
5 = almost complete understanding

|  | My Understanding | |
|---|---|---|
|  | **After Training** | **Before Training** |
| How would you describe your understanding of the following? | None<br>Little<br>Moderate<br>Quite a bit<br>Complete | None<br>Little<br>Moderate<br>Quite a bit<br>Complete |
| 1. The financial pressures faced by low-income families in meeting basic needs | 1<br>2<br>3<br>4<br>5 | 1<br>2<br>3<br>4<br>5 |
| 2. The difficult choices people with low-resources need to make each month when stretching limited income | 1<br>2<br>3<br>4<br>5 | 1<br>2<br>3<br>4<br>5 |
| 3. The difficulties in improving one's situation and becoming self-sufficient on a limited income | 1<br>2<br>3<br>4<br>5 | 1<br>2<br>3<br>4<br>5 |
| 4. The emotional stresses and frustrations created by having limited resources | 1<br>2<br>3<br>4<br>5 | 1<br>2<br>3<br>4<br>5 |
| 5. The positive and negative impacts of helpers on people with limited resources | 1<br>2<br>3<br>4<br>5 | 1<br>2<br>3<br>4<br>5 |

# *FAMILY DYNAMICS*

# Fathers and Daughters: A Needed Course in Family Studies

## Linda Nielsen

**ABSTRACT.** Father-daughter relationships should receive more attention in family studies courses. A review of the literature shows that fathers have a lifelong impact on their daughters, yet receive too little attention from educators, mental health and social service workers, and researchers. Especially in families where the parents are unhappily married or divorced, father-daughter relationships need more attention from professionals working with families. By offering a course on Fathers and Daughters similar to the one described in this article, faculty can help students recognize their own biases and misconceptions about fathers, become familiar with recent research and its practical applications in working with fathers and daughters, and often create more meaningful relationships with their own fathers. This college course incorporates a unique variety of teaching techniques: student interviews with their fathers, the completion of more than fifty self-assessment questionnaires, tests that require application of research, critiques of Web sites, and assigned questions that encourage more focused class discussions. *[Article copies available for a fee from The Haworth Document Delivery Service: 1-800-HAWORTH. E-mail address: <docdelivery@haworthpress.com> Website: <http://www.HaworthPress.com> © 2005 by The Haworth Press, Inc. All rights reserved.]*

**KEYWORDS.** Fathers and daughters, father-daughter course, father-daughter relationships, teaching, family studies

---

Linda Nielsen is affiliated with Wake Forest University.

Address correspondence to: Linda Nielsen, Box 7266, Wake Forest University, Winston Salem, NC 27109 (E-mail: nielsen@wfu.edu).

© 2005 by The Haworth Press, Inc. All rights reserved.
doi:10.1300/J002v38n03_01

## INTRODUCTION

Family studies courses are a powerful force in shaping the attitudes and behavior of social and mental health professionals and, as such, need to focus more on father-daughter relationships. While many colleges offer courses devoted exclusively to mother-daughter relationships, almost none offer courses exclusively focused on father-daughter relationships. Moreover, it is difficult to present a balanced, accurate portrait of families when research and college textbooks tend to focus more on father-son and mother-daughter relationships than on fathers and daughters—and even then, focus more on the father's shortcomings than his strengths (Booth & Crouter, 1998; Dienhart, 1998; Griswold, 1998; Lamb, 1997; Pruett, 1999).

Few mental health practitioners and social service workers are well prepared to work with fathers and daughters. Consequently, professionals working with families often pay less attention to fathers' relationships with the children than to mothers' relationships—especially when the children are daughters (Baker & McMurray, 1998; Beale, 1999; Carr, 1998; Fagan & Hawkins, 2003; Long, 1997; Phares, 1999; Walters, 1997). Excluding or ignoring fathers is even more likely when the parents are divorced (Amato & Booth, 1997; Brott, 1999; Nielsen, 1999; Warshak, 2002).

The reason for father-daughter relationships receiving less attention in both research and practice can be traced to the early part of the twentieth century when there was growing concern about the loss of "manliness" in our society. Throughout the 1950s, concerns over boys' becoming too feminine as a result of being raised by overly protective mothers led to fathers being urged to become more involved with their sons in an effort to enhance the "manhood" in the next generation of men (Bederman, 1995; Griswold, 1993). But as we will soon see, the idea that fathers are more important and more necessary to their sons than to their daughters has not altogether disappeared.

Father-daughter relationships merit more attention in the curriculum as we can see by examining these three questions: What is the status of most father-daughter relationships today? How does the parents' unhappy marriage or divorce affect fathers' relationships with their daughters differently than with their sons? And how do daughters benefit from a meaningful, loving, communicative relationship with their fathers?

## FATHER-DAUGHTER RELATIONSHIPS: HOW GOOD, HOW BAD?

The good news is that most married fathers are spending more time than married fathers in previous generations with their children. On average, married, employed fathers spend a little over two hours each weekday and six hours on weekends with their children, while married employed mothers–80 percent of whom spend less time at work and less time commuting than their husbands–spend a little over 3 hours each weekday and 8 hours on weekends with the children (Galinsky, 1999; Milke, 2004). And the more hours the mother works outside the home, the more hours the father generally spends with the kids (Bonney, Kelley, & Levant, 1999; Brayfield, 2003; Crouter, Bumpus, Head, & McHale, 2001).

But the bad news is that fathers still tend to spend more time with their sons (Lamb, 1997; Phares, 1999; Pleck, 1997; Updegraff, McHale, Crouter, & Kupanoff, 2001). Dads also tend to talk more, share more and give more advice to their sons (Hosley & Montemayor, 1997; Larson & Richards, 1994; Shulman & Krenke, 1996; Snarey, 1993). If fathers feel that they are less important or less necessary to their daughters than to their sons, it might help to explain why only 30 percent of the fathers in a recent survey believed that their active involvement in their daughter's life was "vital" to her health and well being (Roper Poll, 2004). Or why, when adults were asked what gender they would prefer *if they could only have one child*, most men said sons and most women said daughters (Dahl & Moretti, 2004). Likewise, 80 percent of adoptive parents request a girl mainly because the driving force in most adoptions is the wife (Pertman, 2000).

The good news is that the majority of fathers and daughters say they love one another and get along well most of the time. Even during the teenage years, fathers and daughters usually argue less than mothers and daughters–and have a less competitive, more affectionate relationship than fathers and sons (Nielsen, 1996; Shulman & Krenke, 1996; Snarey, 1993). Unfortunately, though, *throughout their lifetimes* daughters and fathers generally do not communicate as comfortably, spend as much time with each other, feel as close to each other emotionally, or get to know one another as well, or talk about as many personal things as mothers and daughters (Amato & Booth, 1997; Lamb, 1997; Nielsen, 1996, 2004; Way & Gillman, 2000). While bonds between mothers and children usually grow stronger over time, those between fathers and children usually do not (Bengston & Roberts, 2002). In short, most fathers and daughters are not getting as much as they could from their relationship.

## UNHAPPY MARRIAGES AND DIVORCE

Father-daughter relationships also merit more attention because, generally speaking, they are more easily damaged than father-son relationships when the parents are unhappily married or divorced. Because mothers and daughters tend to be closer and to confide more in each other, daughters are more likely than sons to turn against dad and form an alliance with mom when things are not going well in the marriage. And if the daughter becomes her unhappy mother's friend, counselor, and confidant, the father-daughter relationship usually suffers (Booth & Crouter, 1998; Cummings & O'Reilly, 1997; Jacobvitz & Bush, 1996). Given this, it is not surprising that father-daughter relationships are usually more damaged than father-son relationships when the parents divorce (Ahrons, 2004; Fabricius, 2003; Hetherington, 2003).

## BENEFITS OF POSITIVE FATHER-DAUGHTER RELATIONSHIPS

Unless students in family studies courses gain a better understanding of fathers' lifelong impact on their daughters lives, they cannot function as effectively in their future professional roles working with families. Our students need to know that fathers generally have as much *or more* impact than mothers do on many aspects of their daughters' lives. For example, the father has the greater impact on the daughters' ability to trust, enjoy, and relate well to the males in her life (Erickson, 1998; Kast, 1997; Leonard, 1998). And daughters who have experienced good fathering are usually more self confident, more self-reliant, and more successful in school and in their careers than daughters who have experienced poor fathering. (Lamb, 1997; Morgan & Wilcoxon, 1998; Perkins, 2001). Daughters with loving, comfortable, communicative relationships with their fathers are also less likely to develop eating disorders (Botta & Dumlao, 2002; Maine, 2004). In short, a father's impact on his daughter's life is far reaching and lifelong.

## THE COURSE DESIGN

### Course Goals

The Fathers and Daughters course has four main goals. These are: (1) to familiarize students with current research and statistics relevant to father-daughter relationships; (2) to show students how to apply the research in practical ways; (3) to recognize their own biases that might limit their effectiveness as professionals; and (4) to motivate them to change some aspect of their relationships with their fathers.

The course is divided into seven major segments. They are as follows: (1) stereotypes, negative beliefs and unfounded assumptions about men that limit or damage father-daughter relationships; (2) the ways in which the father's work, issues related to money, and the daughter's school and career decisions affect the father-daughter relationship; (3) effective and ineffective ways of communicating between fathers and daughters; (4) ways in which daughters can get to know their fathers on a more meaningful, more adult, more honest level; (5) the impact of mothers on father-daughter relationships; (6) ways to deal better with issues related to sex, dating, and marriage that create tension between most fathers and daughters; and, (7) how divorce and remarriage affect the father-daughter relationship and ways to deal with problematic issues and situations.

### Reading Assignments, Grading, Format

The students are required to read *Embracing your father* (Nielsen, 2004), *Throwaway dads* (Parke & Brott, 1999), *Cutting loose* (Halpern, 1990), and selected chapters from *Working fathers* (Levine & Pitinsky, 1998) and *Men can't hear what women don't say* (Farrell, 2000). The grade is based on two written tests, three papers based on interviews with their fathers, seminar participation, and the completion of fifty written questionnaires from *Embracing your father*.

The class is conducted as a seminar and enrollment is limited to sixteen students. The class meets once a week for two and a half hours. This lengthy block of time enables the instructor to use the first hour to focus on research data and still have 80 minutes to discuss the personal implications and applications of the data. The course assignments and activities, however, can also be used with larger classes or in courses where the students meet several times a week for shorter periods of time. To keep the discussion focused, students are required to prepare answers every week to these two questions: (1) What research or ideas surprised or upset you in the assigned reading? Why? (2) What information in this week's reading was most relevant for understanding your relationship with your father or for explaining father-daughter relationships in general? The students then share their answers during class discussion.

## *Media and Web Sites*

Instead of lectures, various media are used to convey and to personalize the research: *Father-Daughter Relationships*–a one hour interview with me and my responses to listeners for National Public Radio (Stasio, 2004), the Academy Award winning animated film *Father and Daughter* (Dudok De Wit, 2000), and the documentaries *Fathers Juggling Families and Work* (Lipschutz & Rosenblatt, 1999), *All Men Are Sons* (Badalamet, 2002), *Going Home: Family Triangles* (James, 1990), and *Fathers and Daughters: Journeys of the Heart* (Lerner, 2005).

Web sites also provide students with research and resourceful ideas. Students are required to submit a ten sentence critique of each of these Web sites: Center for Successful Fathering (www.fathering.org), Dads and Daughters (www.dadsanddaughters.org), Father and Child Society (www.fatherandchild.org), Father's Direct (www.fathersdirect.com), National Men's Resource Center (www.menstuff.org), Men's Voices Magazine (www.menweb.org), National Center for Fathering (www.fathers.com), National Fatherhood Initiative (www.fatherhood.org), National Fathers' Resource Center (www.fathers4kids.org), National Practitioners Network for Fathers and Families (www.npnff.org), and Divorced Fathers Network (www.divorcedfathers.com).

## *Interviewing Their Fathers*

The most powerful assignments are the three interviews with their biological fathers. Fewer than five percent of the students have relationships with their fathers that are so distant or so damaged that they are unable to do these interviews. I create alternative assignments for those students. For example, if the student no longer has any contact with her physically abusive father, she might do a research paper on the effects of physical abuse on children. Or if she has never known her father, she might do a research paper on the effects of father absence.

For the 95 percent of students who are able to conduct the interviews, after the first class each student mails her father the list of 150 questions that she will be asking him in three separate interviews during the semester. Also included in the mailing is an explanation of the assignment as it appears on the course syllabus.

The first interview includes the least personal questions, such as: "What are some of your favorite childhood memories? What kind of relationship did you have with your father? How are you like and unlike each of your parents?" The second interview advances to more personal questions such as: "How do you generally express your anger and how do you usually feel afterwards?" "Tell me about a time when you were unable to forgive someone." The final interview includes the most personal questions, such as: "What are some of the worst decisions you ever made? What do you wish we had more of in our relationship? What are some lessons you learned the hard way? How have your spiritual beliefs changed over time? What do you wish you had known when you were my age?"

The three interviews serve several purposes. Spending time alone with their fathers and asking him questions that have never been asked before can help both to get to know one another on a more meaningful and more adult level. The assignment also provides an opportunity to explore certain topics that have been awkward or impossible for them to discuss in the past. Regardless of how many questions the father is willing to answer or how open he is in answering them, spending several hours talking privately and focusing on the father's life creates an opportunity for more honest, more emotionally intimate communication.

Roughly one third of the students are anxious initially about doing the interviews. This is not surprising, since most fathers and daughters do not spend much time alone discussing anything meaningful or personal. In order to allay their anxieties, the instructor meets with students individually to discuss their concerns and help them prepare for the interviews. Trying to help students overcome their anxieties, however, would not be appropriate in cases where the father had been physically or sexually abusive, or in any other way posed a physical danger to family members.

On average there have been three students a year who are estranged from their fathers for reasons related to their parents' divorce. By meeting individually with these students, the instructor can design a plan for initiating contact with her father. However, this is only an option, if the daughter makes it clear that she wants to renew the relationship with her father and wants the instructor's help in reaching this goal. Although the course is not designed as therapy, the results are therapeutic, especially for those students with the most distant or troubled relationships with their fathers.

## Self-Assessment Quizzes

Students are required to submit 46 written self-assessment quizzes and worksheets from *Embracing your father*. Students are assured that their answers are confidential, although most students choose to share personal information from these assignments in class discussions. Each questionnaire is designed to help students explore their own biases and misconceptions about fathers or to explore their own family relationships. Further details on the classroom activities, assignments, weekly calendar, and test questions are available in *Embracing your father* and the accompanying instructor's manual (Nielsen, 2004).

## SAMPLE AND METHODS

From 1990-2004, 340 female and 6 male students ages 20-24 have taken the course. Approximately 70 percent were majoring in social sciences and 30 percent were Women's Studies minors. Nearly 85 percent were from white, upper middle class families, and 60 percent from the Southeast. Twenty percent had parents who were divorced.

During the first three weeks of the course students completed fifteen self-assessment quizzes and questionnaires from *Embracing your father*. Nearly 70 percent reported having a "good" relationship with their father, while 30 percent reported a "poor" relationship with him. While only five percent gave their relationships with their mothers the lowest rating possible (1 on a five-point scale), almost 20 percent gave their fathers the lowest rating. Nearly 60 percent said they had a closer, more personal relationship with their mother, communicated better with her, and knew more about her than they knew about their father. Only 10 percent felt they were closer to and communicated better with their father than with their mother. Thirty percent said their relationships with each parent were equal in these respects.

More bad news for fathers and daughters: Throughout childhood and during their college years, nearly 90 percent of the daughters spent more time talking to and being with their mothers than with their fathers–especially private time with just the two of them together. Roughly five percent spent equal time being with and talking to both parents during their college years, while a mere four percent spent more time being with or talking to dad than mom.

With respect to students' expectations in their relationships with their fathers, 80 percent want to communicate better–especially about personal things, 60 percent want to get to know him better and be more open in their relationship, 25 percent want to spend more time together, and 20 percent want their father to treat them more like grown-ups. The topic that most would like to talk comfortably and honestly about is related to something unpleasant going on in the family–or something that happened in the past but still has not been discussed or resolved. These topics include: divorce, ongoing marital unhappiness, alcohol or drug problems, depression, eating disorders, adultery, financial issues, and conflicts with extended family members. A close second is a desire to hear more about their father's experiences or get his advice on personal relationships such as his ideas on what it takes to create a good marriage (or why his marriage ended in divorce), his opinions of her boyfriend, or his feelings about her cohabiting with a man instead of getting married.

Given that the majority of students say they want a more communicative, comfortable, and meaningful relationship with their fathers, their answers on the questionnaires are especially sad. Nearly 40 percent go through their mother to communicate with their father about anything personal or "really important." As they have done throughout childhood, this 40 percent relies on their mother to be the family's communications satellite–beaming messages to dad and deciding which information will and will not be relayed to him about the daughter's life. Only 30 percent of the students tell their fathers as much as they tell their mothers about what's going on in their lives or go to him for as much advice about personal issues. Although 80 percent go to their fathers for advice on non-personal issues such as school or car problems, 50 percent admit they are more open and more honest with their mothers. Only 10 percent are more open and honest with their fathers.

Initially, many students have sexist beliefs and negative misconceptions about men as parents–beliefs that may limit their own relationships as well as limit their effectiveness in their future work with families. For example, on written homework quizzes, half of the students initially believe that fathers are less stressed than employed mothers who are trying to balance work and family–a belief that is not supported by recent research (Levine & Pitinsky, 1998; Parke & Brott, 1999; Milke, 2004). And nearly half initially believe that children benefit most socially, academically and psychologically when the father is the only wage earner and the mother stays home to raise the kids–a belief that is not supported by recent research on employed mothers (Barnett & Rivers, 1996; Geiger, 1996; Lamb, 1997).

## *RESULTS*

The students' comments on the anonymous final course evaluations, the three papers, and their written weekly assignments provide the assessment data for the course. Based on these three sources, 90 percent of the students achieve all four course goals. They become familiar with the most current research, learn how to use the research in applied settings, recognize their personal biases and societal beliefs that may limit their effectiveness as professionals, and change some aspect of the relationship with their own fathers. Moreover, 80 percent of the students earn at least a B on the tests, demonstrating that they have become well acquainted with the research.

The single biggest change is that 82 percent of the students say that their relationships improved and their understanding of father-daughter relationships grew as a consequence of the three interviews with their fathers. Only 10 percent say they "got nothing out of the interviews." Likewise, in their papers nearly 60 percent of the students write about positive changes in how they perceive their fathers. And nearly half write about their growing awareness of the negative impact their mothers have had on certain aspects of their father-daughter relationships.

The students with divorced parents generally experience the biggest changes in terms of how they perceive and how they treat their fathers. Most become more forgiving, understanding, and open minded about events that have harmed their relationship or detracted from it. All of the students who were estranged from their fathers for reasons related to their parents divorce ended up speaking to, or getting together with, their father by the end of the semester.

According to an old maxim, "Nature didn't make us perfect so it did the next best thing by making us blind to our own faults." But as a result of this course, many students become more aware of their own shortcomings as daughters. In their papers nearly 80 percent of the students mention ways in which *they*, not their fathers, have been limiting or preventing the relationship from becoming more meaningful and personal.

## CONCLUSION

By paying more attention to father-daughter relationships in family studies, we provide future professionals with the kind of knowledge and attitudes that will make them more "father friendly" in their careers. By more fully appreciating the lifelong impact that fathers have on their daughters, students will inevitably devote more energy and attention to strengthening father-daughter relationships in their future careers. Students must be made more aware of their own misconceptions and inaccurate information about fathers by becoming acquainted with the most current research on father-daughter relationships.

Although the interviews with their fathers and the self-assessment quizzes have the most powerful impact, the Web site assignments, documentaries, and seminar format also engage and challenge students. By including seminar participation in the final grade and assigning the same two discussion questions for seminars each week, students are refrained from meandering, repeating themselves, or focusing only on personal storytelling. Likewise, creating exam questions that require students to support their answers with references to specific studies, while also demanding that they apply research findings to particular problems, extends test-taking beyond the traditional exercise of merely memorizing facts.

The impact of the course goes beyond preparing students to be more effective in their future professions. Having developed a more accurate and compassionate perspective on fathers and a deeper appreciation for the way our society too often demeans, demoralizes and disenfranchises dads, almost every student ends up with a more comfortable, communicative, meaningful relationship with her own father. It has been said that people would rather have one good soul satisfying *emotion* than consider any of the *facts* when making up their minds about anything important. But in the case of this Fathers and Daughters course, most students *do* change their minds as well as their emotions as a consequence of looking at the facts.

## REFERENCES

Ahrons, C. (2004). *We're still family*. NY: Harper Collins.
Amato, P. & Booth, A. (1997). *Generation at risk*. Cambridge: Harvard University Press.
Badalamet, J. (2002). *All men are sons*. NY: AMAS Films.

Baker, R. & McMurray, A. (1998). Fathers' loss of school involvement. *Journal of Family Issues, 3*, 201-214.
Barnett, R. & Rivers, C. (1996). *She works, he works.* San Francisco: Harper.
Beale, A. (1999). Involving fathers in parent education. *Professional School Counseling, 3*, 5-12.
Bederman, G. (1995). *Manliness and civilization.* University of Chicago.
Bengston, V. B. & Roberts, R. (2002). *How families still matter.* NY: Cambridge University Press.
Bonney, J., Kelley, M., & Levant, R. (1999). Fathers in dual earner families. *Journal of Family Psychology, 13*, 401-415.
Booth, A. & Crouter, A. (1998). *Men in families.* Mahway, NJ: Erlbaum.
Botta, R. & Dumlao, R. (2002). Communication patterns between fathers and daughters and eating disorders. *Health Communications, 14*, 199-219.
Brayfield, A. (2003). Juggling jobs and kids. *Journal of Marriage and the Family, 57*, 321-332.
Brott, A. (1999). *Single father.* NY: Abbeville Press.
Carr, A. (1998). Including fathers in family therapy. *Contemporary Family Therapy, 20*, 371-383.
Crouter, A., Bumpus, M., Head, M., & McHale, S. (2001). Employment and child care. *Journal of Early Adolescence, 10*, 296-312.
Cummings, M. & O'Reilly, A. (1997). Effects of marital quality. In M. Lamb (Ed.), *The role of the father in child development* (pp. 49-65). NY: Wiley.
Dahl, G. & Moretti, E. (2004). *The demand for sons.* Cambridge, MA: National Bureau of Economic Research.
Dienhart, A. (1998). *Reshaping fatherhood.* Thousand Oaks, CA: Sage.
Dudok De Wit, M. (2000). *Father and daughter.* Hollywood, CA: Acme Filmworks.
Erickson, B. (1998). *Longing for dad.* Deerfield Beach, FL: Health Communications.
Fabricius, W. (2003). Listening to children of divorce. *Family Relations, 52*, 385-396.
Fagan, J. & Hawkins, A. (2003). *Clinical and educational interventions with fathers.* NY: Haworth.
Farrell, W. (2000). *Women can't hear what men don't say.* NY: Putnam.
Galinsky, E. (1999). *Ask the children.* NY: William Morrow.
Geiger, B. (1996). *Fathers as primary caregivers.* NY: Greenwood Press.
Griswold, R. (1993). *Fatherhood in America.* NY: Basic Books.
Griswold, R. (1998). History and politics of fatherlessness. In C. Daniels (Ed.), *Lost fathers.* NY: St. Martin's.
Halpern, H. (1990). *Cutting loose.* NY: Fireside.
Hetherington, M. (2003). *For better or worse.* NY: Norton.
Hosley, C. & Montemayor, R. (1997). Fathers and adolescents. In M. Lamb (Ed.), *The role of the father in child development* (pp. 162-178). NY: Wiley.
Jacobvitz, D. & Bush, N. (1996). Parent child alliances. *Developmental Psychology, 32*, 732-743.
James, R. (1990). *Going home: A family systems view of change.* NY: AMES Films.
Kast, V. (1997). *Father-daughter, mother-son.* Rockport, Mass: Element.
Lamb, M. (1997). *The role of the father in child development.* NY: Wiley.

Larson, R. & Richards, M. (1994). *Divergent realities: Emotional lives of mothers, fathers and adolescents*. NY: Basic Books.
Leonard, L. (1998). *The wounded woman: Healing the father daughter wound*. Boston: Shambala.
Lerner, H. (2005). *Fathers and daughters: Journeys of the heart*. NY: Creative Expansions Films.
Levine, J. & Pitinsky, T. (1998). *Working fathers*. Reading, MA: Addison Wesley.
Lipschutz, M. & Rosenblatt, R. (1999). *Fathers juggling family and work*. NY: The Fatherhood Project.
Long, N. (1997). Are we contributing to the devaluation of fathers? *Clinical Child Psychology & Psychiatry, 2*, 197-200.
Maine, M. (2004). *Father hunger: The impact of fathers on daughters*. NY: Gurze Books.
Milke, M. (2004). The time squeeze. *Journal of Marriage and the Family, 66*, 739-761.
Morgan, J. & Wilcoxon, A. (1998). Fathers and daughters. *Family Therapy, 25*, 73-84.
Nielsen, L. (1996). *Adolescence: A contemporary view*. Ft. Worth, TX: Harcourt Brace.
Nielsen, L. (1999). Demeaning, demoralizing and disenfranchising divorced dads. *Journal of Divorce & Remarriage, 31*, 139-177.
Nielsen, L. (2004). *Embracing your father: How to build the relationship you've always wanted with your dad*. NY: McGraw Hill.
Parke, R. & Brott, A. (1999). *Throwaway dads*. NY: Houghton Mifflin.
Perkins, R. (2001). Father-daughter relationships and family interactions. *College Student Journal, 35*, 616-626.
Pertman, A. (2000). *Adoption nation*. NY: Basic Books.
Phares, V. (1999). *Poppa psychology*. Westport, CT: Praeger.
Pleck, J. (1997). Paternal involvement. In M. Lamb (Ed.), *The role of the father in child development* (pp. 66-104). NY: Wiley.
Pruett, K. (1999). *Fatherneed*. Boston: Free Press.
Roper Poll. (2004). *Dads talk about their daughters*. NY: United Business Media.
Shulman, S. & Krenke, I. (1996). *Fathers and adolescents*. NY: Routledge.
Snarey, J. (1993). *How fathers care for the next generation*. Cambridge, MA: Harvard University.
Stasio, F. (2004). *Fathers and daughters*. Chapel Hill, NC: National Public Radio.
Updegraff, K., McHale, S., Crouter, A., & Kupanoff, K. (2001). Parents' involvement in adolescent peer relationships. *Journal of Marriage and the Family, 63*, 655-668.
Walters, J. (1997). Talking with fathers. *Clinical Child Psychology & Psychiatry, 2*, 197-199.
Warshak, R. (2002). *Divorce poison*. NY: Regan Books.
Way, N. & Gillman, D. (2000). Adolescent girls' perceptions of their relationships with their fathers. *Journal of Early Adolescence, 20*, 309-331.

# Service-Learning in Parenting Education: Insights from Students and Parent Participants

Rhonda A. Richardson
Audrey Kraynak
Maureen Blankemeyer
Kathleen A. Walker

**ABSTRACT.** The field of family studies is particularly suited to service-learning, but one area that has not received much attention in this regard is that of parenting education. This article highlights a series of parenting education workshops that were incorporated into a parent-child relationships course, utilizing a developmental assets framework. Student reflections and parent evaluations are used to consider the extent to which the service-learning activity enabled students to apply course content to real-world experiences, view themselves as emerging professionals, and have a positive impact on the community. Implications for continuing or replicating similar service learning experiences are included. *[Article copies available for a fee from The Haworth Document Delivery Service: 1-800-HAWORTH. E-mail address: <docdelivery@haworthpress.com> Website: <http://www.HaworthPress.com> © 2005 by The Haworth Press, Inc. All rights reserved.]*

---

Rhonda A. Richardson, Audrey Kraynak, Maureen Blankemeyer, and Kathleen A. Walker are affiliated with the School of Family and Consumer Studies, Kent State University.

Address correspondence to: Rhonda A. Richardson, PhD, CFLE, School of Family and Consumer Studies, 100 Nixson Hall, Kent State University, Kent, OH 44242 (E-mail: rrichard@kent.edu).

An earlier version of this paper was presented at the annual meeting of the National Council on Family Relations, Vancouver, BC, November 2003.

© 2005 by The Haworth Press, Inc. All rights reserved.
doi:10.1300/J002v38n03_02

**KEYWORDS.** Developmental assets, parent-child relationships, parenting education, service-learning

## INTRODUCTION

Increasingly, colleges and universities are encouraging collaboration between academia and the community in the form of service-learning partnerships. Service-learning has been defined as "a form of experiential learning in which students participate in an authentic service activity that helps meet needs identified by the community" (Eby, 2001, p. 2). Students benefit from this hands-on experience because it allows them to connect theory and practice. Concurrently, the citizens of the community benefit from the students' efforts to prevent and solve social problems.

The field of family studies is particularly suited to service-learning because of its applied, interactive, and ecological perspective (Leach, 1998). In fact, some would argue that family studies has always been engaged in community collaboration; it is merely the label "service-learning" that is new (Paulins, 1999). Recently, special issues of family science journals (e.g., *Kappa Omicron Nu* and *Journal of Teaching in Marriage and Family*) and journals of higher education (e.g., *College Student Journal*) have highlighted articles describing human development and family science courses that incorporate service-learning as an integral part of the curriculum. The content of these courses focuses on developmental dysfunction, divorce and remarriage (Ritblatt & Obegi, 2001), child development (Conner, 2004; Strage, 2004), children's language and family literacy (Clawson & Couse, 2002), independent living skills for at-risk youth, and gerontology (Hamon & Way, 2001; Jarrott, 2001; Karasik & Berke, 2001). In order to assess student outcomes of the service-learning component, most of these courses included the requirement that students reflect on their experiences. Such reflections are critical elements of service-learning because they facilitate the understanding, use, and transfer of knowledge from experience (Giles & Eyler, 1994), as well as promote changes in attitudes (Myers-Lipton, 1996). In addition, they provide students and faculty with a way to evaluate whether or not the objectives of the service-learning experience were met.

Although a variety of family studies courses are represented in the service-learning literature, one area that has been given very little attention is parenting education. A few service-learning parenting education projects are in progress (Spoth, Greenberg, Bierman, & Redmond, 2004; Warner, 2000), yet very little is known about the student outcomes of service-learning in parenting education. Our study addresses this gap in the literature.

The purpose of this article is to introduce college and university instructors and community partners to a service-learning project that was implemented in a parenting education course. The project, which was based on the developmental assets framework, was initiated in order to help students experience the real world applicability of their course content. Additional outcomes of this service-learning activity included helping students view themselves as emerging professionals in the field of family studies and giving them an opportunity to have a positive impact on their community. In addition to highlighting the parenting education service-learning project, this article also provides a description of students' reflections and workshop participants' evaluations as a means of assessing the effectiveness of the service-learning experience. Finally, implications for continuing or replicating similar service-learning experiences in the area of parenting education are included.

## CONCEPTUAL FRAMEWORK FOR PARENTING EDUCATION WORKSHOPS

Parenting education has been defined as "any conscious and organized effort to provide parents with information, skills, experiences or resources intended to strengthen, improve or enrich their performance in the parenting role" (Myers-Walls & Myers-Bowman, 1999, p. 71). Whether aimed at treatment of existing problems, prevention of anticipated problems, or enrichment of problem-free conditions, the ultimate goal of parenting education generally is to facilitate parent behaviors that will influence positive developmental outcomes in children (Smith, Perou, & Lesesne, 2002).

In developing the present service-learning activity, faculty identified a framework to guide the students' work and to organize the individual workshop sessions into one overall theme. The framework selected for this purpose was the Search Institute's forty developmental assets (Benson, Galbraith & Espeland, 1998). This framework was chosen because its theoretical underpinnings are consistent with the course content in our Human Development and Family Studies curriculum and because it allows for versatility in selecting topics and targeting audiences for parenting education workshops. Specifically, ecological systems theory underlies the developmental assets approach, recognizing that it is not just families but also schools, religious groups or organizations, and communities that have a role to play in helping children acquire what they need to succeed (Benson et al., 1998). Furthermore, the developmental assets approach is based on a positive, strengths-based perspective and can be used for either prevention of problems in children at risk or enrichment of existing developmental strengths. Additionally, the developmental assets framework covers a wide range of topics, from family communication to school engagement to self-esteem enhancement. Educators can choose which developmental assets to emphasize based on the needs of their target audience and the assets can be adapted to parents of children of diverse ages (Leffert, Benson, & Roehlkepartain, 1997). The groundwork for the developmental assets approach was laid by Benson's (1993) report of the results of a nationwide survey of youth perspectives, values and behaviors. The current model describes forty assets that Benson and his associates at the Search Institute have identified as protective mechanisms or qualities that "help youth lead productive healthy lives" (Benson et al., 1998, p. 3). Youth who possessed 31 or more of these assets exhibited more positive behaviors than other youth and engaged in fewer problem behaviors such as chemical abuse, early sexual activity or school problems. However, the Search Institute found that sixth through twelfth grade students typically had only 18 of these assets (Benson et al., 1998). Recent research examining developmental assets in relation to a variety of youth outcomes such as tobacco use (Atkins, Oman, Vesely, Aspy, & McLeroy, 2002), eating disorders, (French, Leffert, Story, Neumark-Sztainer, Hannan, & Benson, 2001), and suicide attempts (Price, Dake, & Kucharewski, 2001) lends further support to the conclusion that it is imperative for parents and communities to examine how many of these assets their youth possess and seek ways to augment current practices that promote the acquisition of these building blocks for healthy development.

According to Benson and colleagues, the protective characteristics and skills that comprise the developmental assets model are divided into four categories of external assets and four categories of internal assets. External assets are those "things in a young person's environment (home, school, and community) that support, nurture, and empower him or her, set boundaries and expectations, and make constructive use of his or her time" (Benson et al., 1998, p. 4). The four types of external assets include support, empowerment, boundaries and expectations, and constructive use of time. Internal assets are those "attitudes, values, and competencies that belong in the head and heart of every child" (p. 5). They include commitment to learning, positive values, social competencies, and positive identity. Each external and internal sub category is composed of four to six characteristics.

## PARENTING EDUCATION WORKSHOPS AS A SERVICE-LEARNING ACTIVITY

For the present service-learning activity, students in the Human Development and Family Studies program at a large Midwestern state university used the developmental assets approach as the basis for conducting parenting workshops in a number of local communities. This service-learning activity was launched when a local children's behavioral health care agency contracted with the university's Human Development and Family Studies program to offer parenting education to all of the elementary and middle schools in the county. Faculty decided to incorporate the activity into an existing senior-level course entitled Parent-Child Relationships.

The initial parenting education workshops consisted of a series of one-hour sessions delivered to parents in each of ten different school districts. As this parenting education initiative evolved, efforts concentrated on providing multiple sessions in single school districts and on utilizing the versatility of the developmental assets approach to address a variety of topics of interest to parents. Specific developmental assets used in programming included "helping your child avoid harm" and "helping your child be a good person and friend."

Over three semesters, 93 students presented 20 workshops to a total of 113 parents at elementary and middle schools throughout the county. Working in groups of four or five, students selected several of the forty developmental assets on which to base their workshop session. They were provided 30 minutes of class time on a weekly basis to convene their groups and work on their respective projects, although much of the planning and organization for each workshop took place outside of the classroom. The presentations incorporated a variety of teaching techniques such as Power Point presentations, skits, interactive activities, and parent discussions of issues pertaining to the assets. The presentations were supported with handouts developed by the students. Parents were invited via school newsletters and flyers to attend the workshops, which were scheduled for weekday evenings in their child's school library or gymnasium. Free child care was provided to facilitate parent attendance.

Student reflections on their experiences and parent evaluations of the workshops were used to assess the effectiveness of the service-learning activity. Of primary interest was whether or not students were able to: (a) apply course content to their real-world experiences, (b) view themselves as emerging professionals in the field of family studies, and (c) have a positive impact on their community.

## STUDENT REFLECTIONS

After the conclusion of the workshops, students were asked to reflect on their experiences regarding the parenting education sessions. Specifically, they were asked what they learned about themselves and what they learned about delivering parenting education. Given the similarity of the students' reflective pieces from the three semesters, their written responses were combined and qualitatively analyzed for the present study (Patton, 1990). Themes were identified and exemplars were selected to illustrate each theme.

### What Students Learned About Themselves

Five major themes emerged from the students' answers concerning what they learned about themselves. These themes were categorized as: (a) intrapersonal issues, (b) concerns or fears related to delivering parenting education, (c) knowledge about the developmental assets framework, (d) insights into group work, and (e) clarification of future career plans.

*Intrapersonal Issues.* As might be expected, the theme of intrapersonal issues was very common among students' reflections regarding what they learned about themselves. Students became aware of strengths they previously did not know they had. One student stated, "I ... learned that being creative is something that I really value and need." Another student said, "I learned that I can take on leadership roles. With this project, I really spoke up for myself and took charge." The students also described changes in their confidence levels, most often related to speaking in front of groups. One student wrote, "It was once extremely hard for me to speak in public. Now, after practicing with my group, I am much more confident than when we started."

*Concerns and Fears.* A second theme centered on concerns and fears related to delivering parenting education information. Although many of the students identified an increase in their confidence levels, many of them also described their nervousness related to public speaking. One student wrote, "I don't know if I am really ready to go out and make presentations like the one that we did. I felt nervous through the whole presentation." Another one stated, "I . . . learned that I need more opportunities and experiences with talking in front of people. I feel I get too nervous and worry too much."

*Knowledge of the Developmental Assets Framework.* Students also demonstrated their knowledge of the developmental assets framework when reflecting on what they learned about themselves. One student who indicated she learned she had 35 of the developmental assets identified by the Search Institute wrote, "My parents did a great job in raising me, for me to have so many assets." Another student wrote, "One of the things I learned was that if I had done what we recommend to the parents from commitment to learning [a group of developmental assets], I would have been better able to have enjoyed school and homework. I want to do these ideas with my children."

*Insights into Group Work.* Not surprisingly, a fourth theme centered on the students' insights into group work. One student said, "I learned that it is difficult to work in groups, but helpful to get different viewpoints." Another student wrote, "I . . . learned that I work well in groups, but I would almost rather do everything by myself. It was nice to have the support of the group members, but sometimes I like when things are done my way." One student stated, "I have worked on group projects before and it is not my favorite type of course work, [but] with this group, I learned how to enjoy myself and to let go."

*Clarification of Their Future Career Plans.* Another theme that emerged from the students' reflections on what they learned about themselves focused on the clarification of their future career plans. Some of the students indicated they wanted parenting education to be a part of their future careers. One student wrote, "I learned that I really enjoy doing parent education. It is a very rewarding feeling to be able to take what I have learned and use the knowledge to help others." Other students suggested that parenting education was not the career choice for them. One student said, "I learned that this is not the type of profession I am looking for. Although I did well and it was a good learning experience, it made me realize that I want to work with youth even more than I did before."

## What Students Learned About Delivering Parenting Education

Six themes emerged from the students' answers concerning what they learned about delivering parenting education. These included: (a) the importance of parenting education for children and parents, (b) the lack of participation in parenting education (i.e., low attendance at workshops), (c) the eagerness and willingness of parents to learn, (d) concerns about not being taken seriously as parent educators since they were not parents themselves, (e) the developmental assets content in parenting education, and (f) parenting education methodology.

Students frequently commented on the importance of parenting education. One student wrote, "Parent education is very important. Also, parent education can really turn someone's life around." Another student stated, "Parents need . . . education. They need to come to the presentations and learn about their child's competencies and developmental assets."

Many of the students expressed concerns about what they perceived as a lack of parental participation in parenting education. One student stated, "Unfortunately, I saw that many parents are not interested in learning new ideas to become better or more effective parents. The turnout of parents was low and I wish more parents would take advantage of the opportunity to learn." Another one wrote, "I learned that parent education is a tough thing to provide. I was surprised at the small attendance we had at the presentations. I thought more parents would come."

In spite of low parent turnout, many students also gained insight into the eagerness and willingness of parents to learn. As stated by one student, "Parents are willing to learn to be the best parents that they can possibly be. Before I thought that parents wanted to do things their way and not take any advice from anyone else." Another student explained, "Parents are receptive to the information you are telling them. They are really interested in information you have to offer and are willing to talk about their experiences if you ask them."

Some students gained insight into concerns about not being taken seriously as parent educators since they were not parents themselves. For example, one student wrote, "One thing I learned about parenting education is that it is hard to try and teach parents when I don't have any [children]. In a way I felt weird giving them information when they are the ones with children and the ones with experience." Another student reflected that he/she had reached a different conclusion: "One thing is that you should not be intimidated by teaching someone that is older and more experienced than you."

Students also identified the developmental assets content as an important part of what they learned about parenting education. One student wrote, "[I learned] parents need to stress the value of school and homework to their child. Make sure, as parents, you are available to help your child with school work and give advice about school when needed." Another student stated, "One thing I learned about parent education is that every child needs some if not all of the developmental assets."

A sixth and final theme that emerged from the students' reflections on parenting education was related to methodology. Students stated they learned how to deliver parenting education effectively. Many of them indicated the material must be relevant to parents. One student suggested, "*If the topic is relevant to their lives, they [parents] are very receptive.*" Students also discussed the importance of a knowledgeable and well-prepared presenter. One student wrote, "The parent education session taught me that parents really do listen if they know you are a qualified individual with tangible information that applies to their circumstances." Other students mentioned specific strategies to use when providing parent education. One student stated, "I . . . found when working with parents it is important to break things down so they can understand what point you are trying to make. Providing examples to them seems to be very effective in getting the point across."

The students' reflections demonstrated the success of the service-learning activity in meeting its first objective of enabling students to experience the real world applicability of their course content. Students clearly were able to apply course content (i.e., knowledge of the developmental assets) to real-world experiences (i.e., providing parenting workshops). Students' retention of the content of the developmental assets model was enhanced through teaching it to their fellow students and to the parents who attended the workshop. In addition, the developmental assets content became both personally and professionally meaningful to the students as they reflected on their own childhood experiences and received confirmation and feedback from the parents attending the workshops. In essence, this approach provided both a preventative and an intervention focus–prevention for the students in their future role as parents and intervention for the parents as they evolved in this role.

The service-learning activity also presented students with the opportunity to better understand the process of parenting. Specifically, the workshops changed students' perceptions of parents. Students cited the parents' willingness to learn and their receptivity to the information presented helped students to view the parents in a more positive way.

Student reflections indicated that the second objective of the service-learning activity also was met. That is, they began to view themselves as emerging professionals and reflected on the reality involved in delivering parenting education while taking pleasure in helping parents improve the lives of their children. Additionally, the service-learning project helped a number of students clarify career plans. Some found parenting education rewarding, while others realized they preferred working with a different population, such as adolescents or preschoolers.

Because the delivery format for these workshops involved small groups, the students were guided through the process of becoming a team as well as delivering a successful presentation. They learned to accept different viewpoints and to accommodate and cooperate in order to reach the goal of effectively delivering the content for their workshop, a worthy learning experience for future professionals who will collaborate with other service providers in order to meet the needs of those they serve.

## PARENT EVALUATIONS

The third objective (for students to have a positive impact on their community) was assessed using the participating parents' evaluations of the student-led workshops. Program effectiveness was evaluated in each of the three semesters the service-learning activity was conducted. The evaluation process evolved based on learning from previous semesters. Thus, both formative and summative evaluations were used in this course.

### *Semester One*

Parents in the first semester of student-led workshops completed a 4-item assessment of their knowledge of developmental assets prior to the beginning of each presentation. At the conclusion of the presentation, the assessment was re-administered along with an evaluation of the effectiveness of the presentation. Students were given copies of the evaluation results to assist them in reflecting on their strengths and limitations as parenting educators. Results of the pre-test and post-test evaluations indicated a notable increase in parental knowledge about developmental assets as a result of attending the presentation. Before attending the presentation, only 20% of parents could name two developmental assets, while 100% were able to do so following the presentation. Prior to the presentation 33% of parents indicated that they understood what developmental assets were, and after the presentation 100% indicated an understanding. Similarly, the percentage of parents who understood why developmental assets are important increased from 40% at pre-test to 100% at post-test. There was also a marked increase in parents' knowledge of ways to help children build assets, from 40% at pre-test to 100% at post-test. Furthermore, 98% of the parents indicated that they learned something new from the presentation, and 96% indicated that they would recommend the presentation to other parents.

*Semester Two*

During the second semester workshop series, parents again completed a pretest prior to the first workshop session to assess their knowledge of developmental assets. Results, which were shared with students as a source of feedback, indicated that the majority of parents (66%) had a moderate level of knowledge prior to participation in the workshop. At the conclusion of each of the four workshop sessions, parents completed a post-test developed by the students that assessed their understanding of the developmental assets presented in that evening's workshop.

In addition, parents were asked to describe "the two most important things learned today." Results suggested that at each session parents gained additional knowledge regarding the developmental assets model. For example, in reflecting on the session about the external asset "support," parents reported learning the importance of (a) having another adult to whom the child could talk, (b) encouraging the child to participate in activities but not too many, (c) maintaining eye contact with the child when talking to them, and (d) being aware of body language.

*Semester Three*

For the third semester workshop series, students again participated in developing the evaluation component of the workshops. At the conclusion of the weekly session, parents completed a two-part evaluation questionnaire. Part 1 of this questionnaire consisted of six multiple-choice questions that were developed by the respective student presenters to assess knowledge of the content covered during that evening's session. Part 2 was a 12-item evaluation of the workshop format and delivery, including clarity and usefulness of information, knowledge level of presenters, and diversity of workshop activities. Results of the evaluations indicated that upon completion of each session, the majority of parents were able to correctly answer most questions pertaining to that evening's developmental assets topics and were "satisfied" to "very satisfied" with all components of the workshops. In addition to answering the content-related questions and indicating the degree of satisfaction, parents were asked two open-ended questions at the conclusion of each workshop. One, what were the two most important things you learned this evening? Two, what is one thing you already knew that was reaffirmed this evening? Finally, in an effort to evaluate transfer of learning from the workshop to the home, sessions 2-6 began with a weekly update and feedback from the parents regarding any reflections about the previous topics and application of information. Specifically, they indicated the frequency with which they found themselves thinking about or using information from the parenting workshop over the past week. In addition, parents provided an example of a time when they thought about or used information from the parenting enrichment workshop. Parent responses indicated that every week each parent thought about and used information from the parenting session at least a few times.

Each semester's parent evaluations confirmed that students were making a positive impact on their community (objective three of the service-learning activity). Program evaluation measures indicated that even affluent, highly educated parents benefited from the workshops as indicated by enhanced knowledge of the developmental assets concept. Moreover, these parents wanted to discuss child rearing issues and sought input from other parents. The workshops allowed the parents to build a support network and receive affirmation and validation regarding their parenting practices. Parental feedback also suggested that beginning each session with a time to reflect on the previous session and discuss how they had applied the information helped to reinforce and clarify the information presented.

## *IMPLICATIONS*

The students' reflections on their experiences illustrate favorable outcomes that result from participating in service-learning in parenting education. This is consistent with studies of service-learning outcomes in other family studies courses (Conner, 2004; Karasik & Berke, 2001; Ritblatt & Obegi, 2001). As discussed previously, these guided experiences using the developmental assets model benefited students in a number of areas. Intrapersonally, students developed an enhanced self-awareness of individual strengths and limitations, such as leadership skills as well as increased self-confidence regarding public presentations. Moreover, many students recognized that the anxiety that they felt was also experienced by their classmates, thus lending a quality of normalcy to the experience.

Although this service-learning project provided a number of benefits to the students enrolled in the parent-child relationship course, there were ancillary benefits for the academic program as well. For example, the service-learning project provided opportunities for curriculum refinement. The course instructors were able to learn about parents' concerns and tailor the content so that it was relevant to the parents' needs. In addition, the instructors were able to help students deliver the content using a variety of activities and materials so that the concepts were easily understood by the parents. Utilizing information from the students' reflections, the instructors provided class discussions and problem solving sessions that focused on such issues as the misperception that low attendance was solely due to parental apathy. Other class discussions/problem solving could focus on (a) how best to market the program, and, (b) how to overcome the obstacles that limit parental attendance (i.e., parents' schedule constraints and lack of child care arrangements).

In addition to refining the curriculum with respect to student learning, the student reflections and parent feedback prompted discussions among the authors of this manuscript about how requirements of other courses in the major could be adapted to facilitate the success of the service-learning project. Consequently, one of the authors, who teaches the Child Development course, required that students attend the parenting education workshops to both provide child care and to observe the students who would be delivering parenting education. This may have resolved some parents' difficulty with attending the workshops due to lack of child care. In addition, this collaboration provided the Child Development students with an idea of what to expect when they take the senior-level parenting course. It also gave them valuable practical experience and helped to explain the theories of Erikson, Piaget, and Bronfenbrenner.

Each semester, evaluations from parents proved helpful in encouraging students to perceive themselves as contributing professionals. The transition from student to professional is a process that can begin before graduation with hands-on service-learning activities. Furthermore, exposing students to formal evaluations, however limited, helps students to better understand the connection between research and practice. Future research could help determine if students exposed to evaluation in service-learning are more amenable to undertaking evaluation projects as part of their professional roles.

## LOGISTICAL CONSIDERATIONS

Whenever a new project is implemented, there are logistical considerations that may interfere with achieving a successful outcome. In discussing the use of service-learning in family studies, Karasik and Berke (2001) identified the lack of community support as one potential barrier. Without strong campus-community relationships it may be difficult to convince parents to attend student-led parenting education workshops. Issues of time, energy and creativity on the part of both faculty and students also need to be addressed (Karasik & Berke, 2001; Ritblatt & Obegi, 2001). Additional specific barriers may include funding limitations, faculty workloads, delegating organizational responsibilities, site locations, availability of child care, and the commitment of participants. The discussion that follows addresses each of these barriers.

This service-learning project was made possible by a grant from a local children's behavioral health agency which provided a stipend to the instructor and allowed purchasing of supplies and equipment (i.e., a video camera that was used to record the presentations). The video tapes were used by the students to evaluate themselves and by the instructors to provide actual examples to the successive Parent-Child Relationship classes. Although the grant funding has expired, faculty in the Human Development and Family Studies program felt strongly about the beneficial aspects of this service-learning project and have continued to incorporate it into the course curriculum.

This service-learning project added a concomitant responsibility to that of teaching the course content. Consequently, the faculty workload was adjusted to reflect this additional responsibility. Also, facilitation of the service-learning activity has been recognized as service to the community when evaluating faculty scholarship within our Human Development and Family Studies program.

As the service-learning project evolved, various approaches to managing the logistics of workshop registration and attendance emerged. For example, during the second semester of providing parenting education in a local school district, the registration process, provision of food, details regarding the site, and arrangements for the high school students who provided child care were handled by the Parent Teacher Organization president. However, in semesters one and three, the course instructor managed the registration and details concerning the site. In semester three, child care arrangements were handled by the instructor who assigned students enrolled in the Child Development class to provide child care, thus eliminating a potential barrier to parental attendance at the workshops.

Perhaps the greatest obstacle for this service-learning project was the inconsistent attendance. During all three semesters, the workshops were held in the evening with the intent of accommodating working parents. However, perhaps parents were too busy to come to workshops at night. Therefore, weekend sessions may be more attractive to potential enrollees. Even when there was a formal registration prior to the beginning of the workshops, as occurred in the second semester, it was difficult to know how many parents would attend each week. In spite of flyers and reminder postcards, low parental attendance during the third semester remained a source of concern. Therefore, it may be necessary to offer some sort of incentive or reward for attending sessions. For example, enticing parents by providing dinner or gift certificates donated by local merchants may encourage greater parental commitment to attending the student-led workshops. Furthermore, attendance may be enhanced by consistently offering the sessions in one location. This may enable parents in the community to recognize and remember the program and to market it via word of mouth. Although our workshops were held in school buildings, other community facilities may be available, including local churches or libraries that provide space without charging a fee.

## *SUMMARY*

This article described the use of the developmental assets approach as a fundamental component of a parenting education service-learning project. The approach's breadth and versatility make it an ideal choice as a framework for parenting education workshops provided by service-learners—our students. This framework benefited the community, helping parents become more aware of behaviors or assets that lead to positive child developmental outcomes. Parents learned from the students, but students also learned from the parents, as evidenced by their written reflections. Students were given the opportunity to apply course content to real-world experiences and began to see themselves as emerging professionals.

As is apparent in the descriptions of the three semesters' workshops, service-learning, as with any course requirement, warrants careful monitoring and revision as deemed appropriate. This article suggests that feedback from multiple sources is essential for continually adapting and improving the service-learning component of a course. For the present project, parents, course instructors and their colleagues, and students all provided valuable insights that were used throughout the evolution of the service-learning project. Others who choose to incorporate service-learning into their curricula are encouraged to utilize feedback from multiple sources, including the home, school, and community.

Continued exploration of what students, parents, and instructors bring to the service-learning experience are needed, but based on the numerous benefits identified by students as well as the implications for curriculum refinement and development, service-learning is likely to continue to be an important component of family studies courses. This is particularly relevant for those courses that focus on parenting education. It is our hope that the description of this experience will encourage others to incorporate service-learning opportunities in their parenting classes. We believe that these opportunities provide valuable benefits for students as they discover what being a parent educator really entails.

## REFERENCES

Atkins, L. A., Oman, R. F., Vesely, S. K., Aspy, C. B., & McLeroy, K. (2002). Adolescent tobacco use: The protective effects of developmental assets. *American Journal of Health Promotion, 14*, 198-205.

Benson, P. L. (1993). *The troubled journey: A portrait of 6th-12th grade youth.* Minneapolis, MN: Search Institute.

Benson, P. L., Galbraith, J., & Espeland, P. (1998). *What kids need to succeed.* Minneapolis, MN: Free Spirit.

Clawson, M. A. & Couse, L. J. (2002). Using service-learning in academic courses. *Kappa Omicron Nu FORUM, 13*, 61-74.

Conner, D. B. (2004). The effects of course-related service projects in a child development course. *College Student Journal, 38*, 462-471.

Eby, J. W. (2001). The promise of service-learning for family science: An overview. *Journal of Teaching in Marriage and Family, 1*, 1-13.
French, S. A., Leffert, N., Story, M., Neumark-Sztainer, D., Hannan, P., & Benson, P. L. (2001). Adolescent binge/purge and weight loss behaviors: Associations with developmental assets. *Journal of Adolescent Health, 28*, 211-221.
Giles, D. & Eyler, J. (1994). The impact of a college community service laboratory on students' personal, social, and cognitive outcomes. *Journal of Adolescence, 17*, 327-339.
Hamon, R. R. & Way, C. E. (2001). Integrating intergenerational service-learning into the family science curriculum. *Journal of Teaching in Marriage and Family, 1*, 65-83.
Jarrott, S. E. (2001). Service-learning at dementia care programs: A social history project. *Journal of Teaching in Marriage and Family, 1*, 1-12.
Karasik, R. J. & Berke, D. L. (2001). Classroom and community: Experiential education in family studies and gerontology. *Journal of Teaching in Marriage and Family, 1*, 13-38.
Leach, L. J. (1998). Teaching resource management while modeling community: An experience in service-learning in a family and consumer sciences course. *Kappa Omicron Nu FORUM, 10*, 19-27.
Leffert, N., Benson, P. L., & Roehlkepartain, J. L. (1997). *Starting out right: Developmental assets for children*. Minneapolis, MN: Search Institute.
Myers-Lipton, S. J. (1996). Effects of service-learning on college students' attitudes toward international understanding. *Journal of College Student Development, 37*, 659-688.
Myers-Walls, J. A. & Myers-Bowman, K. S. (1999). Sorting through parent education resources: Values and the example of socially conscious parenting. *Family Science Review, 12*, 69-86.
Patton, M. Q. (1990). *Qualitative evaluation and research methods*. Newbury Park, CA: Sage Publications.
Paulins, V. A. (1999). Service-learning and civic responsibility: The consumer in American society. *Journal of Family & Consumer Sciences, 91*, 66-72.
Price, J. H., Dake, J. A., & Kucharewski, R. (2001). Assets as predictors of suicide attempts in African American inner-city youths. *American Journal of Health Behavior, 25*, 367-375.
Ritblatt, S. N. & Obegi, A. D. (2001). Community-based service-learning in the family sciences: Course development and learning outcomes. *Journal of Teaching in Marriage and Family, 1*, 45-64.
Smith, C., Perou, R., & Lesesne, C. (2002). Parent education. In M. H. Bornstein (Ed.), *Handbook of parenting, vol 4: Social conditions and applied parenting* (pp. 389-410). Mahwah, NJ: Lawrence Erlbaum Associates.
Spoth, R., Greenberg, M., Bierman, K., & Redmond, C. (2004). PROSPER Community-university partnership model for public education systems: Capacity building for evidence-based, competence-building prevention. *Prevention Science, 5*, 31-39.
Strage, A. (2004). Long-term academic benefits of service-learning: When and where do they manifest themselves? *College Student Journal, 38*, 257-261.
Warner, L. (2000). University students and parents together: Expanding undergraduates' experiential base. *Early Childhood Education Journal, 27*, 227-233.

#  Teaching About International Families Across the United States

Mihaela Robila
Alan C. Taylor

**ABSTRACT.** Due to increasing globalization, teaching students about international families is important in preparing them to become competent multicultural educators. This study assessed the current existence of family studies courses across the United States which focus on international families. More than 110 undergraduate and 76 graduate family science/studies programs were reviewed. However, only 20 undergraduate and 10 graduate courses on international families or cross-cultural perspectives on families were identified. Recommendations are provided for including this type of course in family studies curricula, and several textbooks on international families are suggested. *[Article copies available for a fee from The Haworth Document Delivery Service: 1-800-HAWORTH. E-mail address: <docdelivery@haworthpress.com> Website: <http://www.HaworthPress.com> © 2005 by The Haworth Press, Inc. All rights reserved.]*

**KEYWORDS.** Family studies courses, international families, teaching

---

Mihaela Robila is affiliated with Queens College, City University of New York. Alan C. Taylor is affiliated with Syracuse University.

Address correspondence to: Mihaela Robila, PhD, CFLE, Assistant Professor in Family Science, 306 Remsen Hall, Queens College, CUNY, 65-30 Kissena Boulevard, Flushing, NY 11367 (E-mail: mrobila@qc.edu).

## INTRODUCTION

Culture influences all aspects of human life, including values, assumptions, beliefs, and practices (Arnett, 2002). The influence of culture becomes much more complex in an interdependent and interconnected world where modern technology, travel, human migration, multinational economic developments, and other globalization trends have blurred borders between cultures (Fountin, 1995; Lim & Renshaw, 2001). The increasing interconnectedness and intermingling of cultures as a result of globalization requires that pedagogies concerning diversity focus on creating new knowledge and meanings about changing cultures (Banks, 2001; Germain, 1998; Lim & Renshaw, 2001). While students who travel or study abroad may experience first hand other cultures and families, those without such opportunities often fail to acquire new knowledge and gain meaningful experiences with diverse cultures. For students without these experiences, it is mandatory that they be provided with a curriculum that offers courses on cultural diversity and/or international issues.

The adjustment of the educational system to the needs of current society is imperative. Research has assessed the role of multicultural education in preparing students to face the challenges of the world (Roopnarine & Gielen, 2004). How universities approach multicultural education and integrate it into their curricula is an indicator of the value placed on its importance. Gay and Fox (1995) describe four themes regarding the theory and philosophy of multicultural education: (1) the importance of contextual and developmental appropriateness in making decisions about educational reforms to promote ethnic and cultural diversity (relationship between formal institutional policies and practices, informal expectations); (2) the implementation of multicultural education requires systematic and systemic change (purposeful planning, regularity of occurrence); (3) the integral role of personal values, beliefs, and life experiences in teaching and learning processes; and, (4) multicultural education is transformative and revolutionary (advocates cooperative plurality).

It is desirable for multicultural education to be included in all departments, and not limited solely to anthropology or cultural studies programs (Arnett, 2002; Comunian & Gielen, 2001). The increasing complexity of family matters (e.g., structure) in recent decades has contributed to the growth of family studies as a field and the increase in family studies programs throughout the country.

Given the rapid rate of globalization, teaching about international families by using a cross-cultural approach becomes increasingly important (Roopnarine & Gielen, 2004). Understanding complex family issues from an international perspective prepares students to work more effectively with scholars and families from other cultures. By establishing May 13th as the Day of International Families and celebrating the 10th Anniversary of the Year of the Family in 2004, the United Nations recognized the importance of understanding families in a multicultural world. By learning how families are affected by social, economic, and political forces, scholars can better identify ways to help families adapt and live fulfilling lives.

As part of the global community, organizations in the United States have played an active role in promoting the well being of international families by creating and supporting family programs, and by organizing conferences and seminars on family issues (i.e., National Council on Family Relations, International Family Strengths Conferences). Such activities demand professionals well-trained in cultural diversity and family functioning in different societies. Universities and family studies programs need to produce more scholars who are prepared to fulfill these roles. More specifically, the way programs organize their curricula to include courses such as Teaching about International Families become critical factors in the students' educational experience and professional development.

As in other fields, family studies has to reflect the needs of the modern world. Further, as people travel more frequently and become involved in various international programs, understanding more about the world's families becomes an important tool of diplomacy. Educating family studies students about global issues helps produce competent professionals ready to tackle the current issues of society. Courses on teaching about international families as well as teaching about ethnic diversity should be part of a program's core requirements to ensure the exposure of all students to issues of cultural diversity. There is a need for family studies programs to introduce students to other cultures, while attempting to instill feelings of acceptance, and tolerance of differences, as there is little doubt they will be exposed to people of all types and nationalities in the workforce.

Although there is some literature on multicultural education (e.g., Bennett, 2003; Gollnick, 2002; Lantis & Kuzma, 2000; Pang, 2001), the research on teaching about international families appears to be extremely limited. The goal of this article is twofold: One, to examine the current status of family studies courses at universities in the United

States that focus on international families. And two, to identify and highlight textbooks that might prove useful in teaching about international families.

## *METHODS*

### *Procedure*

In conducting our review of programs we began with the *"Graduate and Undergraduate Study in Marriage and Family: A guide to Bachelor's, Master's, and Doctoral Programs in the United States and Canada"* edited by Jason D. Hans (2002). While the guide contains information about 235 family programs in the United States and Canada, this study focuses only on programs in the United States. The publication includes reviews of various departments, including family studies, family therapy, family and consumer sciences, psychology, counseling, and sociology. The author of the guide contacts university administrators and requested specific information about their programs including the courses they offer (Hans, 2002). Updated every three years, it represents perhaps the most comprehensive listing of undergraduate and graduate programs in the field of family studies.

The next step was to identify course titles in family studies/science programs that indicated international/cross-cultural content specifically. Courses focused on "international families" include such terms as marital relations, gender roles, and parenting in families in other countries. We defined the term "cross-culturalism" to be synonymous with the idea of going across cultures, which is not the same as courses focusing on the variation/diversity within a certain culture. Therefore, for recording purposes, courses with "international/cross-culturalism" within their titles were grouped separately from those focusing on the diversity within a specific culture (e.g., courses on ethnicity, race, or gender).

After reviewing a list of study areas provided by departments of universities, those identified as family science/studies were selected (Hans, 2002). Examples included, "Child and Family Studies," Child and Family Development," "Family and Consumer Sciences," "Family and Community," "Family Development," "Family and Human Services," "Family Studies," "Human Development and Family Studies," and "Family Life Education." The study included 110 undergraduate and 76 graduate programs.

## Data Analysis

The comparative method of analysis (Miles & Huberman, 1994; Strauss & Corbin, 1990) was used to examine the data. The courses were compared for similarities and differences and both major categories and subcategories were created (Strauss & Corbin, 1990). The two main categories created were international families and cross cultural perspectives on families (courses that focused on international families), and cultural diversity (courses that focused on general diversity within United States or on specific ethnic groups). Descriptions and syllabi of courses that covered international families were examined for their content.

## RESULTS

### Undergraduate Courses

Using the criteria described above, 111 undergraduate programs were identified as offering courses on international families and cultural diversity. Of those, 54 (48%) programs offer some type of cultural diversity course. Because some programs offer more than one course on cultural diversity, a total of 74 courses on related topics were identified. Of these 74, two types of courses were identified: the first focused on cross-cultural/global context/international issues and families. The second centered on ethnic identity/race/diversity. Only 20 courses (18%) were offered specifically on cross-cultural/international issues, with a mere six course titles reflecting some global/international content (see Table 1).

Few courses were offered specifically on the topic of international/cross-cultural/global perspectives and families. Another category included courses on diversity. In some cases, the courses focused directly on "cultural diversity," while others addressed "diversity" more indirectly. By offering courses specifically on international families, students are given the opportunity to gain more in-depth knowledge about families in different cultural settings. It also helps to create awareness among students that not all families have similar experiences, which is essential to developing cultural sensitivity. Within the diversity/ethnicity category, some courses focused on race and ethnicity/minorities in general, while others focused on a single ethnic group, such as African American or Latino. There was no course offered on Asian

TABLE 1. Undergraduate Courses Offered on Cultural Diversity

| Category | Sub-Category | Number of Courses | Examples of Undergraduate Courses |
|---|---|---|---|
| International Families/Cross-Cultural Perspectives on Families | International Families and Children | 4 | "The Family in International Settings" "International Approaches to Child Advocacy" "International Families" |
| | Cross-Cultural Perspectives on Families | 14 | "The Child and Family in Cross-Cultural Perspective" "Family in Cross-Cultural Perspectives" "Cross-Cultural Family Patterns" "Family Diversity Across Cultures" "Family Life Education Across Cultures" |
| | Global Context/ Multicultural | 6 | "Marriage and Family in a Global Context" "Global and Diverse Families" "Multicultural Families" "Family Stress and Coping: Multicultural Focus" |
| Cultural Diversity/ Diversity Within United States | Diversity | 19 | "Family Diversity" "Families and Cultural Diversity" |
| | Ethnicity/Race | 19 | "Human Services and Family Ethnicity" "Ethnic Identity and Awareness in Children and Families" |
| | Black/African American | 9 | "Black American Family Patterns" "Black Families" |
| | Latinos | 3 | "Latina/Latino Families and Children in the United States" "Latinos" |

American families. A third category included courses that address family diversity within the United States.

## *Graduate Courses*

Seventy-six graduate programs, identified by the criteria described above, offered courses on international families. As presented in Table 2, 29 programs (38%) offered 39 courses on cultural diversity. Of the 29 graduate programs, 18 (62%) also offered courses on cultural diversity at the undergraduate level. Only five course titles were found to focus exclusively on international families. Examples of the courses offered are provided in Table 2.

TABLE 2. Graduate Courses Offered on Cultural Diversity

| Category | Sub-Category | Number of Courses | Examples of Courses |
|---|---|---|---|
| International Families/Cross-Cultural Perspectives on Families | International Families | 5 | "International Home Economics" "History of Family in Russia" "International Approaches to Child Advocacy" |
| | Cross-Cultural Perspectives | 5 | "Cross-Cultural Perspectives" "Childhood and Family in Cross-Cultural Perspectives" "Human Development in Cross-Cultural Perspectives" |
| Cultural Diversity/ Diversity Within United States | Diversity | 10 | "Cultural Influences on Children and Families" "Culturally Diverse Family Systems" "Diversity in Individuals and Families" |
| | Ethnicity | 1 | "Advanced Seminar in Multi-Cultural Families" |
| | General | 15 | "Ethnic Families" "Gender and Minorities Across the Lifespan" "Gender and Ethnicity" |
| | Black/African American | 3 | "The Afro-American Family" "Development of Black Children and Their Families: Research and Policy" |

A review of the descriptions and syllabi for undergraduate and graduate courses on international families revealed several common themes; these syllabi were obtained based on internet searches using keywords similar to the ones used to identify the original courses. All the courses aimed to provide an overview of family dynamics in different cultures. Among the processes explored were marital functioning, gender roles, and child rearing beliefs and strategies. The courses were also designed to give students the opportunity to appreciate the roles of political, socio-economic, and cultural influences in human and family development. With respect to course objectives, students are expected to acquire a broad understanding of culture, understand specific theories on human and family development, explore contemporary methodologies used in the study of families across cultures, analyze the link between family processes and family outcomes in different cultures, and discuss policies employed by different societies which affect families and children.

## DISCUSSION

The results of the study indicate that the number of courses offered on cultural diversity is relatively small, with more than half of the undergraduate programs not offering a single class on diversity. Surprisingly, the number of graduate courses on cultural diversity is even smaller, with less than 40% of the departments offering courses on cultural diversity. Furthermore, very few graduate programs offer courses on international families. This could be the result of the lack of textbooks on international families until recently which hindered the development of courses on families in different countries.

### Strengths and Limitations

This study has several unique and important strengths. First, it is perhaps the first study that explored course offerings on cultural diversity in graduate and undergraduate family studies programs. Second, by reviewing programs in several areas related to family sciences (such as family studies, family services, family life education) a considerable assortment of programs was identified. And third, studying a representative sample of many colleges and university programs around the nation provided a more comprehensive look at the current situation in the family studies field.

When discussing the results of this study, certain limitations have to be considered. The "Guide of Graduate and Undergraduate Programs in Marriage and Family" contains information on a limited number of programs. There may be programs in existence that offer courses on cross-culturalism/international families and related topics that are not included in the guide Also, not having syllabi for all of the courses identified made it difficult to evaluate their content; given the extension of Blackboard (and similar tools) it is increasingly likely that syllabi will no longer be available online. In addition, some courses on international families might have been missed under the unspecified umbrella of "advanced topics" or "seminars." However, listing a course under this category suggests that the course, although offered, is not offered regularly. It is recommended that as the number of courses of this type increases, the textbooks, activities, learning materials, and teaching techniques be evaluated.

## Recommendations

Curriculum changes are necessary if we want to promote multicultural education in family studies departments. Many of the programs reviewed prepare future teachers and are therefore influential with respect to long-term educational practices. Often, graduating students in these programs enter K-12 classrooms and other educational settings as teachers, promoting, or sometimes not promoting, cultural diversity awareness (Gay & Fox, 1995). Graduates entering the workforce who have had the opportunity to take courses centered on multicultural education will be better equipped with the skills and knowledge to interact with and understand the dynamics of immigrant families residing in the U.S. For example, social service professionals assigned to an immigrant family will be a step ahead if they are aware of the cultural specifics of that family. Also, family life educators teaching community parenting and marriage education classes will be more sensitive to the dynamics of other cultures if they have been taught about diversity in their university courses.

The offering of introductory courses as well as more advanced or more specialized courses (e.g., focused on parenting or policies in different countries) would be beneficial. There is an urgent need to introduce this type of course in the curricula, particularly at the graduate level. Graduates of masters and doctoral programs in family studies have considerable opportunities and a profound responsibility to be knowledgeable proponents of cultural diversity.

We recommend including courses on cultural diversity, not only as optional electives, but also as core course requirements for family science programs. In addition, we recommend emphasizing the study of international families as a part of the requirements under the first content area–family diversity–for the Certification of Family Life Educators (CFLE) sponsored by the National Council on Family Relations (NCFR) (Bredehoft & Cassidy, 1995). If the NCFR CFLE program were to emphasize the benefits of courses on international families, it might motivate family studies programs to include these types of courses in their curriculum.

Offering courses on cultural diversity is not enough to ensure a thorough cultural education, however. Multicultural competence is emerging as a defining feature in professional development, training, and education (Sue, Bingham, & Vasquez, 1999). Thus, courses should include meaningful instructional methods, such as a focus on affective learning, personal involvement, and giving voice to multiple social realities (Gay & Fox, 1995). It is not enough that students learn about families in different cultures; they must also understand the personal and social value of this knowledge (Banks, 1994; Gay & Fox, 1995). Teaching strategies should legitimize the voices and experiences of different ethnic and cultural groups, and provide students with opportunities to examine their feelings about issues of cultural diversity (Gay & Fox, 1995). Courses on international families should also teach students to be reflective, critical thinkers, and decision makers, and to promote social justice (Darling-Hammond, French, & Garcia-Lopez, 2002; Gay, 1994; Van Soest & Garcia, 2003). The courses which are currently being offered may already utilize these pedagogies; this would be an area of study for future research.

As family scholars and teachers strive to educate and influence others through community programming (e.g., parenting classes), there is a growing need for professionals to understand and show sensitivity to the cultural context of the population they teach. As the U.S. population continues to become increasingly diverse, family scholars will likely encounter many people from distinctive ethnic and cultural backgrounds (Dilg, 1999; Forehand & Kotchick, 1996; Kailin, 2002). Courses on multicultural diversity should address the unique cultural contributions and potential barriers to effective family programs (e.g., parent training) future family educators may encounter. It is only through an awareness of, and an appreciation for, the diversity of cultures that family scholars will achieve their goal of helping families live life to its fullest potential within the context of their particular culture, as well as within the umbrella culture of society at large (Forehand & Kotchick, 1996).

## TEXTBOOKS FOR TEACHING ABOUT INTERNATIONAL FAMILIES

A challenge for any course instructor is finding appropriate textbooks to meet the demands of the desired course objectives. An additional goal of this paper was to identify a handful of appropriate textbooks that may be employed in courses studying international families and relationships. To examine current family relationships and human development from around the world, we have identified textbooks that seem to provide appropriate research and content from a true international perspective.

Elaine Leeder's (2004) book, *The Family in Global Perspective: A Gendered Journey*, examines the continually changing faces of family life in western countries and contrasts them with the lives of families in parts of Africa, Asia and Latin America. By first comparing the history of the family from various parts of the globe, Leeder looks at the impact of globalization on family structure; gendered behavior; intergenerational relationships; and relationship dissolution.

Jaipaul Roopnarine and Uwe Gielen (2004) edited *Families in Global Perspective*, which examines 14 different cultures from around the globe and their respective family dynamics. Some of the cultures examined include China, Indonesia, Egypt, Turkey, Brazil and South Africa. The authors address multiple family topics from these cultures, including such areas as gender socialization, parent-child relationships, marriage and mating, and division of household labor, among others.

In *Lives Across Cultures: Cross Cultural Human Development* (Gardiner, Mutter, & Kosmitzki, 1998), basic principles and research findings are connected to practical everyday situations that take place in diverse cultures throughout the world. The authors present global research in the area of social settings (family, school and culture) and the activities occurring within them (social interactions, personality development, and cognitive change). As opposed to covering families from different international communities, each chapter focuses on social settings and activities and then discusses the international research surrounding them.

Robila's (2004) edited book, *Families in Eastern Europe*, examines family patterns and changes in 14 countries in Eastern Europe (e.g., Bulgaria, Czech Republic, Hungary, Lithuania, Macedonia, Poland, Romania, Russia). The authors of each chapter explain family processes in each particular country, focusing on the historic, social and economic contexts and the impact they have on families. The book provides demographic information about families and discusses cultural traditions, marital and gender roles, parenting processes, family policy and a sampling of programs within each society.

*International Perspectives on Family Violence and Abuse: A Cognitive Ecological Approach*, an edited book by Malley-Morrison (2004), addresses the question of domestic violence and its culturally specific definitions in various areas around the world. Chapters include cultural and historical experiences that contribute to differences and similarities in the perspectives on family violence held by citizens of different countries.

Hamon and Ingoldsby's (2003) *Mate Selection Across Cultures* provides a contemporary, global perspective on the couple formation process in various regions of the world, including Ecuador, Kenya, Israel, Spain, and others. The chapters underline the variation that exists within any one country and also reviews such concepts as modernization/traditionalism, arranged marriage/free choice, love/family practicality, cohabitation/marriage, and collectivism/individualism.

While our initial attempts to find appropriate textbooks examining international families seemed difficult, it was refreshing to discover several new textbooks recently published which will fill that void. We are hopeful that additional authors will realize the necessity of textbooks on cross-cultural topics and compile relevant current research into a textbook format, so that instructors will have many choices for a text. Finally, we believe that with the increased production of such texts, family science departments will be more apt to introduce courses on international families, cultural diversity, and related topics. Such courses are necessary in the preparation of family science specialists who will be confronting a rapidly changing world.

## REFERENCES

Arnett, J. J. (2002). The psychology of globalization. *American Psychologist, 57*, 774-783.

Banks, J. A. (1994). *An introduction to multicultural education*. Boston: Allyn and Bacon. Banks, J. A. (2001). *Cultural diversity and education: Foundations, curriculum and teaching*. Needham Heights, MA: Pearson Education Company.

Bennett, C. (2003). *Comprehensive multicultural education: Theory and practice*. Boston: Allyn and Bacon.

Bredehoft, D. & Cassidy, D. (Eds.). (1995). College and university curriculum guidelines in Family Life Education. Minnesota: National Council on Family Relations. Retrieved 6-22-05 from http://www.ncfr.org/pdf/FLE_Substance_Areas.pdf

Comunian, A. & Gielen, U. (Eds.). (2001). *International perspectives on human development*. Lengerich, Germany: Pabst.

Darling-Hammond, L., French, J., & Garcia-Lopez, M. (2002). *Learning to teach for social justice*. New York: Teachers College Press.

Dilg, M. (1999). *Race and culture in the classroom: Teaching and learning through multicultural education*. Boston: Allyn and Bacon.

Forehand, R. & Kotchick, B. A. (1996). Cultural diversity: A wake-up call for parent training. *Behavior Therapy, 27*, 187-206.

Fountin, S. (1995). *Education for development: A teacher's source for global learning*. Portsmouth, NH: Heinemann.

Gardiner, H. W., Mutter, J. D., & Kosmitzki, C. (1998). *Lives across cultures: Cross-cultural human development.* Boston: Allyn and Bacon.
Gay, G. (1994). *At the essence of learning: Multicultural education.* West Lafayette, IN: Kappa Delta Phi.
Gay, G. & Fox, W. (1995). The cultural ethos of the academy: Potentials and perils for multicultural education reform. In S. Jackson & J. Solis (Eds.), *Beyond the comfort zones in multiculturalism: Confronting the politics of privilege* (pp. 239-257). Westport, CT: Bergin & Garvey.
Germain, M. H. (1998). *Worldly teachers: Cultural learning and pedagogy.* Westport, CT: Bergin & Garvey.
Gollnick, D. M. (2002). *Multicultural education in a pluralistic society* (6th ed.). Upper Saddle River, NJ: Merrill.
Hamon, R. R. & Ingoldsby, B. (2003). (Eds.). *Mate selection across cultures.* Thousand Oaks, CA: Sage Publications.
Hans, J. D. (2002). *Graduate and undergraduate study in marriage and family: A guide to bachelor's, master's, and doctoral programs in the United States and Canada.* Columbia, MO: Family Scholar Publications.
Kailin, J. (2002). *Antiracist education: From theory to practice.* Lanham, MD: Rowman & Littlefield Publishers.
Lantis, J. S. & Kuzma, L. M. (2000). (Eds.). *The new international studies classroom: Active teaching, active learning.* Boulder, CO: Lynne Rienner Publishers.
Leeder, E. J. (2004). *The family in global perspective: A gendered journey.* Thousand Oaks, CA: Sage Publications.
Lim, L. & Renshaw, P. (2001). The relevance of sociocultural theory to culturally diverse partnerships and communities. *Journal of Child and Family Studies, 10,* 9-21.
Malley-Morrison, K. (2004). *International perspectives on family violence and abuse: A cognitive ecological approach.* Mahwah, NJ: Erlbaum.
Miles, M. B. & Huberman, M. A. (1994). *Qualitative data analysis (2nd ed.).* Thousand Oaks, CA: Sage Publications.
Pang, V. O. (2001). *Multicultural education: A caring-centered, reflective approach.* Boston: McGraw-Hill.
Robila, M. (Ed.). (2004). *Families in Eastern Europe.* Oxford: Elsevier.
Roopnarine, J. L. & Gielen, U. P. (Eds.). (2004). *Families in a global perspective: An introduction.* Boston: Allyn and Bacon.
Strauss, A. & Corbin, J. (1990). *Basics of qualitative research.* Newbury Park, CA: Sage. Publications.
Sue, D. W., Bingham, R. P., & Vasquez, M. (1999). The diversification of psychology: A multicultural revolution. *American Psychologist, 54,* 1061-1069.
Van Soest, D. & Garcia, B. (2003). *Diversity education for social justice: Mastering teaching skills.* Alexandria, VA: Council on Social Work Education.

# International Families in Cross-Cultural Perspective: A Family Strengths Approach

Nilufer P. Medora

**ABSTRACT.** This article presents an overview and suggested guidelines to propose, develop, and teach a course on international families from a family strengths perspective. The course objectives, ground rules, content, readings, requirements, supplemental tools, assessment techniques, and students' evaluation and comments about the course are outlined. Family strengths and key concepts utilized in teaching such a course are examined. Family life among African-Americans, Asian-Americans, and Mexican-Americans is discussed. Also, historical, cultural, social, and political factors influencing mate selection, marriage, parenting, and family life cycle stages in the Hindu and Muslim family are examined. A list of selected audio-visual tools and a sample quiz are also included. *[Article copies available for a fee from The Haworth Document Delivery Service: 1-800-HAWORTH. E-mail address: <docdelivery@haworthpress.com> Website: <http://www.HaworthPress.com> © 2005 by The Haworth Press, Inc. All rights reserved.]*

**KEYWORDS.** Cultural awareness, cultural diversity, ethnic minority families, family strengths, international families, teaching

---

Nilufer P. Medora is Professor and Certified Family Life Educator at California State University.

Address correspondence to: Nilufer P. Medora, Department of Family and Consumer Sciences, California State University, Long Beach, CA 90840 (E-mail: medora@csulb.edu).

© 2005 by The Haworth Press, Inc. All rights reserved.
doi:10.1300/J002v38n03_04

## INTRODUCTION

Today most American universities want to prepare their students to be effective citizens in a global community. In the age of shrinking international boundaries, changing cultural demographics, and a global economy, students should possess an appreciation for cultural heterogeneity and diversity. In order to do this, these academic institutions are developing new international courses or integrating international content into existing courses. Most experts believe that this type of education has as its goal instilling in students a sense of understanding, appreciation, and acceptance of diverse cultures (Seltzer, Frazier, & Ricks, 1995). Although some of the impetus to include cultural diversity stems from external sources such as accrediting agencies and institutions, there is a pressing concern among campus administrators, faculty, students, and potential employers that courses reflect the changing demographic characteristics of the U.S. and of the state in which one lives (Puente et al., 1993).

According to the United States Census Bureau (2000), the ethnic distribution in the U.S. is comprised of 69% Euro-American, 12% African-American, 13% Latino, 4% Asian, 2% Multi-Racial and "Other" category (United States Census Bureau, 2000). Demographers project that by 2050, only half of America's population will consist of Euro-Americans, as the proportion of other racial and ethnic groups is expected to increase. It is projected that the distribution will be 49% Euro-Americans, 25% Latino, 15% African-American, 9% Asian-American and 2% in the "other" category which will include Alaskan, Hawaiian, and those who belong to two or more ethnic groups (Benokraitis, 2002).

In addition to changing demographics internationally and within the U.S., the shrinking of global boundaries, and an increase in the number of immigrants coming to the U.S., educators, researchers, psychologists, family life educators, and family counselors will be required to work with an increasing number of culturally diverse clients. Thus, it is important to understand international clients because many immigrants coming to the U.S. bring their values, beliefs, and customs with them. Even after immigrants have been acculturated into mainstream America, many of their cultural beliefs, traditions, expectations, attitudes, and values continue to be transmitted from generation to generation. The American Counseling Association, the International Association of Couples and Family Counselors and the American Psychological Association have indicated in their codes of ethics that counselors must have taken courses in and be knowledgeable regarding cultural differences to work with ethnically diverse minority U.S. and international clients (American Psychological Association, 1996). The same holds true for certified family life educators. They are required by the National Council on Family Relations to have had coursework on ethnic and international families (Roy & MacDermid, 2003). Therefore, it is of paramount importance for students, educators and researchers to have thorough knowledge and understanding about cultural similarities and differences.

## DEVELOPMENT OF COURSE ON INTERNATIONAL FAMILIES

In response to some of these concerns, it was decided that the undergraduate curriculum in Child Development and Family Studies housed in the Department of Family and Consumer Sciences at California State University, Long Beach (CSULB) would be enhanced if a new class were added to the existing curriculum. This class focused attention on ethnically diverse families within the United States and families in an international context. The new course was entitled "International Families From a Cross-Cultural Perspective: A Family Strengths Approach."

In this course, the Euro-American family is not discussed because the subject is covered in detail in other family studies courses, although indirect references and comparisons are sometimes made (e.g., when family strengths are compared and contrasted). A family strengths perspective (DeFrain, 2003) is employed because the family strengths in different cultures are likely to be varied, unique, and culture-specific. It is important for students to gain insight and understanding about these, because it is hoped that they will develop a greater appreciation, tolerance, and acceptance for the ethnic diversity of their fellow citizens. Thus, when different cultures are discussed, the family strengths that are unique to that particular culture are identified and described.

### *Course Objectives*

Upon completion of this course, the students will be able to achieve the following objectives:

1. Identify family functions, family structural patterns of organization, family forms, kinship and descent rules in selected cultures within and outside the U.S.
2. Describe key concepts relating to race and ethnicity (e.g., racism, ethnocentrism, prejudice, stereotyping, and discrimination).
3. Use a cross-cultural perspective to compare and contrast different values, customs, traditions, beliefs, mores, and behavior patterns in selected cultures as they have implications for individual development and family functioning.
4. Evaluate the impact of geographic, economic, political, social, cultural, and technological factors on individuals and families in international settings.
5. Analyze religious and socio-cultural phenomena such as child-rearing practices, gender roles, rites-of-passage, mate-selection and marriage customs, divorce, kinship expectations, family life cycle patterns, aging, death and dying from a life cycle perspective in selected minority and cross-cultural settings.
6. Assess immigration trends, identify common difficulties, and describe patterns of adjustment and adaptation of ethnic minority families in the U.S.
7. Compare and contrast family strengths cross-nationally and cross-culturally.

## *Ground Rules*

On the first day of class I emphasize that when we delve into family life in other cultures, we will be discussing cultural, social, and religious issues that have affected and influenced people and families living within and outside the U.S. These issues are likely to stir some negative and curious emotional responses to a few of the customs and beliefs, but this is normal and part of the learning process. Organista et al. (2000) provide the following recommendations to employ at the beginning of the semester and to facilitate the presentation of course materials and class discussions:

Inform students that group discussions present a unique opportunity to share and listen to alternative viewpoints in a respectful environment. Students should not personalize the comments being discussed and should not attempt to sway the opinions of fellow class members. Tell students to refrain from pejorative terms, accusatory statements, and inflammatory language in their discussions. Instructors should refrain initially from expressing a definitive viewpoint on a particular discussion topic. Instead, restate questions posed to the instructor by the students for further class discussion. As the instructor, it may also be helpful to model one's struggle in addressing cultural diversity issues (Organista et al., 2000, p. 13).

## Course Content and Issues

It is impossible to cover and do justice to all the different ethnic families in the U.S. or to all the families in the world within a single course. Therefore, over a 16-week semester, the specific families examined in this class are chosen based on the knowledge and expertise of the instructor.

### Section I

Terminology and concepts are introduced in the first section of the course. Some of the terms and concepts appear in book chapters, journal articles, popular periodicals and required course readings. Examples of the terms and concepts discussed include: family forms (e.g., conjugal family, consanguine family, extended family, etc.), rules of residence (patrilocal, matrilocal, ambilocal, etc.), and descent groups (unilineal descent, matrilineal descent, double descent, and forms of marriage). Because most of the citizens in non-western cultures greatly value and emphasize descent groups (Ember & Ember, 2002; Murphy, 1989; Nanda & Warms, 2002; Stanton, 1995), the concepts of lineage, clan, phratry, moiety, and others are discussed and the forms, functions and utility of a descent group are outlined.

One of the greatest challenges when teaching about relevant terminology for this course is to provide an open forum to discuss potentially diverse and emotionally difficult concepts relating to race, ethnicity, culture, discrimination, stereotyping and related concerns (Banks, 1995, 2003; Jackson, 1999; Karp & Sammour, 2000). A majority of the students enrolled in the course acknowledge that they do not have the background, experience, sensitivity, and insight in understanding and discussing families from other cultures in a sensitive, caring, and meaningful manner (Organista et al., 2000).

In order to assist them in the development of their awareness of these subjects, it is important to inform students that recent immigrants, minority students and other citizens still encounter racism in many aspects of their lives. Before they can be sensitive to people from other cultures, the basic concepts of race, racism, ethnic groups, ethnocentrism, minority groups, prejudice, stereotyping, and subtle and covert discrimination are addressed with appropriate examples. Two powerful and educational videos, "The Shadow of Hate" (Teaching Tolerance, 1995) and "Race and Ethnicity" (Bosner, 1991), are used in this section. "The Shadow of Hate" explains the struggle that minority immigrant groups (e.g., Japanese-Americans, Mexican-Americans, Native-American Indians) had to endure to live up to the ideals of liberty, equality, and justice for all. Through documentary footage, viewers are provided a realistic and moving perspective on historical events that occurred in the U.S. The video "Race and Ethnicity" discusses the ills of prejudice and discrimination. Overt and covert discrimination, ethnocentrism, cultural assimilation are defined and explained. These videos act as powerful tools and set the stage for many students to share some of the personal prejudices and discrimination that they had to encounter in their daily lives.

The concept of family strengths is also defined, explained, and revisited throughout the class when different cultures are discussed. There are many different definitions of family strengths. For example, family strengths have been defined as qualities that promote satisfying and fulfilling relationships among family members, and contribute to the family's ability to deal effectively with stress and crises (Medora, Larson, Hortaçsu, & Dave, 2000). Hill (1973) defined family strengths as "those traits that facilitate the ability of the family to meet the needs of its members and the demands made upon it by systems outside the family unit" (p. 3). Since family life is significantly influenced by cultural norms, practices, and beliefs, it follows that family strengths are likely to be culturally based and tend to vary from culture to culture. Therefore, a family strength that is emphasized in one culture may not be viewed positively in another. However, it is important for family science professionals to understand strengths from different cultures so we can best meet the needs of the individuals with whom we work.

## Section II

The second section of the course focuses attention on discussing family life in some of the major ethnic minority groups in the United States (e.g., African-American, Asian-American [Chinese, Japanese, Korean, Vietnamese], Mexican-American, and Jewish cultures). An ethnic minority group has several distinguishing characteristics. It shares a common culture, a historic tradition, and a sense of belonging and peoplehood. It also has unique physical and/or cultural characteristics that enable individuals to identify members easily, often for discriminatory purposes. Ethnic minority groups also tend to be a numerical minority and exercise minimal political and economic power (Banks, 2003). Three cultures will be discussed as examples here: African-American, Asian-American, and Mexican-American.

The following topics are addressed in relationship to the African-American family: (a) the history of migration and slavery, (b) the African-American family under slavery–courtship and marriage, the influence of the extended-kin network, male and female roles in child rearing, and family life patterns during old age, (c) family life of African-Americans after Emancipation, (d) family life during the early 20th century, (e) African-American family of today–the ghetto family and the acculturated middle class African American family–family structure and household composition, the influence of extended-kin network, marriage and parenthood, family life-cycle stages, and sexual roles and, finally, (f) family strengths in African-American families. Examples of African-American family strengths include an ability to perform roles flexibly, a strong religious orientation, and the ability to accept help when appropriate. A video entitled, "Black Is–Black Ain't: A Personal Journey Through Black Identity" (Riggs, 1991) reinforces lecture material about African-American families in historical and contemporary times. This video examines the painful stereotypes that the Euro-Americans have imposed on African-Americans.

When the Asian culture is discussed, the following topics are explained: (a) the history of how and why the first Asians came to the U.S. and an explanation of the different laws and ordinances (e.g., the Foreign Miner's Tax, the Pole Ordinance, the Alien Land Law, Segregation, Immigration, and Employment Laws, etc.) that were enacted to restrict the economic, political, and social advancement of immigrants (Okihiro, 1993), (b) family structure, (c) traditional and contemporary roles of the mother, father, sons and daughters, (d) significance of marriage and marriage customs, (e) cultural beliefs and superstitions, (f) life cycle events, (g) issues of obligation and shaming–saving face (Lee & Zane, 1998; Zhang, 1995), and, (h) communication processes and adaptation and acculturation processes in the U.S.

The video, "Asian-American Cultures in the United States" (Labriola, 1993), further explains how most Americans assume that all Asian cultures are alike but in actuality, there are significant differences and some commonalities. Finally, family strengths in Asian families are identified. Some of the family strengths in Asian families include a sense of familialism over individualism, the interconnection among the individual, family, community, and society, and a sense of respect, obedience and obligation towards the elderly.

The lecture on the Mexican-American family is initiated by introducing and clarifying the origin and connotation of the many different terms that are often used to describe the Mexican-American families–Hispanic, Chicano, Mexican, Latino, and Mexican-American. The following topics are also covered during the lecture: (a) the Mexican migration trends, (b) the Mexican family organization, (c) life cycle events–birth, baptism, quinceañera, marriage, parenthood, old age, the concept of death, dying, and burial practices, (d) the concept of "machismo," (e) the parent-child relationship, (f) child-rearing and socialization practices, (g) sibling relationships, (h) the concept of god parents and compadres, (i) contemporary family life for Mexican-Americans, (j) adaptation patterns and modes of acculturation in the United States, and (k) family strengths of Mexican/Mexican-American families. Some of the family strengths include a commitment to marriage and family, well defined patterns of help and mutual aid among family members, and a strong commitment to religion.

Here a video, "Understanding Our Differences: Mexicans and Americans" (Learning Seed, 1998), examines basic cultural differences that often ignite conflict and mistrust. Recent changes occurring in the Mexican-American family are outlined (e.g., the importance of god parents is waning, higher incidence of divorce, and declining birthrates).

## Section III

In the third section, international families are discussed, including the Hindu, Muslim, and Polynesian (Samoan, New Guinean, Maori) families. The Hindu family and Muslim family are discussed in more detail below.

A brief historical, cultural, and political overview of India is first presented. This is followed by an explanation of religious and ethnic diversity that exists in India. Most people assume that all Indians are followers of Hinduism. Although Hinduism is the dominant religion in India, through the centuries, Indians have learned to coexist with people of other faiths. Thus, while a majority (82.41%) of Indians are Hindu, about 11.67% are Muslims, 2.32% are Christians, 1.99% are Sikhs, .77 are Buddhists, .5% are Jains, Bahais, Jews, Zoarastrains, or other tribal religions (Consulate General of India, n.d.).

In discussing the characteristics of Hindu families, the following topics are covered: (a) the system of castes and sub-castes in the Hindu community, (b) the definition, explanation and benefits of living in a joint family structure, (c) power structure and family controls, (d) major life cycle events, (e) arranged marriages vs. "love marriages," (f) basic requirements for a bride and bridegroom, (g) the dowry system, (h) family life and family values, (i) the status of single and divorced persons in India, (j) salient changes occurring in the contemporary Hindu family, and, (k) important family strengths in the Hindu family. Some of the family strengths of Hindu families include the fact that the joint family provides psychological, economic, and physical support, for all family members including elderly, sick, disabled, divorced, and widowed individuals. The joint family provides built-in playmates for children, tutors, and baby sitters. There is a role hierarchy, and obedience and respect for all elderly individuals are greatly encouraged and emphasized. A slide tape and video clips from a video entitled "India and Her People" (Moyer, 2002) is shown to the students in the class. The media presentation demonstrates highlights about India, explains the contrasts between rural and urban living, and illustrates how the rich and poor live and work. It also discusses the ethnic variations and cultural diversity that exists among the Indian people in all walks of life from the food they eat, the way they dress, to the way they worship.

In discussing the Muslim family, an overview on the fundamentals of Islamic religion and the basic teachings of the prophet Muhammad are introduced. Students are reminded that the Islamic religion can trace its origin in the same way that Christian and Jewish religions can (al Fārūqī & al Fārūqī, 1986; Haddad, 1984; Nasr, 1981). A description of the Muslim world is presented and four basic concepts are incorporated. First, some of the common misconceptions are clarified. For example, most lay people assume that all Muslims are Arabs, and all Arabs are Muslim. However, although the vast majority of the Arabs are Muslim (95%), Arabs account for no more than 20% of the total number of Muslims in the world (Banks, 2003; Hourani, 1991).

Second, the Muslim population of the world is shown on the map of the world. This population now exceeds 1 billion and covers all the continents of the world (Sudo, 1993). Third, a summary of the Prophet Muhammad and the basic precepts of the Qur'an (Koran) are discussed. Finally, the *Five Pillars of Islam* which include (a) the declaration of faith, (b) prayer five times a day, (c) Zakat, (d) fasting, and (e) going on a Hajj (Carolan & Mouton, 2003; Long, 1979; Peters, 1994) are presented. To reinforce these concepts, an *ABC Nightline Special* entitled "The Hajj" that aired on April 18, 1997, is used. In this "special" an

American journalist explains the Islamic faith and then goes to Mecca on a Hajj. The five pillars of Islam are explained and discussed as are the experiences of Muslims when they go on a Hajj to Mecca.

Since there is so much variation among the Muslim families, it would be impossible to cover all the Muslim families. Therefore, the Iranian family is used as an example of a Muslim family in which a brief overview of the historical, religious, cultural, and political events is presented. In addition, the following topics are discussed: (a) the traditional family structure and relationships, (b) power structure and family controls, (c) marriage and child rearing practices, (d) differential treatment of men and women in times of marriage, divorce, and remarriage, (e) life cycle events, (f) death, mourning, and burial practices, (g) three waves of Iranian immigrants that came to the U.S., (h) modes of adaptation in the U.S. such as (i) denigrating the old culture, (ii) denying the new culture, (iii) biculturalism (Jalali, 1996; Ghaffarian, 1987), and finally, (i) family strengths in the Iranian family. Some of the family strengths include a role hierarchy in the family, the belief in assisting the less fortunate and being benevolent and charitable to the community, and living by the precepts of the Koran.

## *Textbook and Other Tools Used for Course Instruction*

A major challenge encountered in teaching this course is finding a textbook that adequately addresses the different ethnic families and international cultures that are outlined in the contents of the course. A packet of readings consisting of book chapters, journal articles, and articles from popular periodicals is used. This packet is constantly updated and current information is incorporated. The course also utilizes a series of guest speakers, videos, and world maps (About Inc., 2005; Central Intelligence Agency, 2005). Quizzes with true or false items that are administered when a new culture is introduced have been developed to assess how much prior knowledge students have about the land, people and family patterns of the culture being addressed. A sample quiz is presented in Table 1.

I have found that a quiz is a good screening device for determining how much knowledge students have about a new culture. It is not graded but students are usually interested in taking it to gauge their general knowledge of the subject matter. Given before a new culture is introduced to the class, I review the correct answers after they have completed the quiz. A small prize, such as a candy bar or box of cookies, is given to the student or students with the highest score.

TABLE 1. Myths and Realities About India and the Hindu Family

Are the following statements Myths (false) or Realities (true)?

1. All Indians are Hindu.  **FALSE**
2. Hindus believe in a multitude of Gods and Goddesses.  **TRUE**
3. Most Hindus are vegetarian; they don't eat meat, chicken, fish, or eggs.  **TRUE**
4. India is the most populated country in the world.  **FALSE**
5. The Hindus believe in and marry within their castes and sub-castes.  **TRUE**
6. Hinduism is older than Christianity and Buddhism.  **TRUE**
7. A religious book of the Hindus is the Bhagwadgita.  **TRUE**
8. Most Indian women get married at the age of 15 years.  **FALSE**
9. India was ruled by Muslim rulers/emperors for almost 300 years.  **TRUE**
10. India is the fifth largest country in the world.  **FALSE**
11. Buddhism was started in India.  **TRUE**
12. A majority of Indians live in the rural areas.  **TRUE**
13. The color of the flag of India is green.  **FALSE**
14. The Hindus do not believe in and practice the dowry system any more.  **FALSE (Dowry has been officially abolished by the government but the practice is still widely followed among Hindus in all the different social classes.)**
15. The practice of having "untouchables" as a separate class is not being practiced in contemporary India.  **FALSE**

Medora, N. P. (2003). India. In J. J. Ponzetti, Jr. (Ed.), *International encyclopedia of marriage and family* (pp. 876-883). New York: Macmillan Reference USA.

## Class Projects and Assignments

As part of the course requirements, the students are expected to complete three multiple-choice exams, a one page research abstract focusing on an international family (other than a Euro-American family) and a critical thinking paper which is a group project. These assignments force many students to go to the library and to consult a variety of different scientific journals, and books that they would not use otherwise.

The abstract is a one-page summary of a research article on an international family published in a scientific journal. The students are instructed to pick any article focusing on international families living outside the U.S. The purpose of this assignment is to ensure that students are knowledgeable and proficient in searching the databases in the library and via the internet, and to understand, interpret, and summarize information in their own words.

A critical application paper is a major course requirement. This assignment requires students to work in a group setting and complete an in-depth study of one specific international culture. The purpose of the critical application paper is to develop research skills, enhance reading, writing, critical thinking skills, and further their abilities to analyze, explain, and synthesize information from books, journals, Websites, popular sources, magazines and periodicals. An important component of this assignment is to ensure that students work cooperatively, productively, and effectively in a group setting. A majority of these students will probably be employed in social service agencies and/or non-profit agencies where they will be required, for the most part, to work with other colleagues on projects. It is hoped that early exposure to working in a group will instill in the students skills to negotiate, work cooperatively, collegially, and assume leadership roles. The students are responsible for forming their own groups of 3 or 4 members. Then, from a list of 15 different international cultures that I have generated, the students pick one culture that they will work on collaboratively as a group.

Each paper is divided into three sections. First, there must be a geographical section that includes a map of the country and surrounding countries/areas. The second section consists of any three of the following events/topics: (a) historical background, (b) birthing practices, (c) childhood and adolescence, (d) rites of passage, (e) mate selection, (f) family structure and functions, (g) stages of the family lifecycle, (h) death, mourning, and burial practices, and (i) beliefs and superstitions.

Finally, the students are required to identify 6-8 of the family strengths for the specific culture that they were assigned. A concluding paragraph summarizes the major findings from each of the three sections of the assigned paper. Sixty percent of the grade is determined by my assessment of the project, while the remaining 40 percent is determined by the students' in-group evaluation of each other's contribution to the project.

## STUDENT DEMOGRAPHICS, COURSE EVALUATION, AND COMMENTS

During the spring of 2003, I taught the course being described with an enrollment of 42 students. The mean age of the students was 22.7 years. Ninety-four percent were women, 88% were seniors, and the remaining 12% were juniors. Thirty-three percent reported their ethnicity as Euro-American, 32% Latino-American, 25% Asian-American, 6% Multi-Racial, and 4% International. Eighty-two percent of the students were Family and Consumer Science majors; the remaining 18% were non-majors from business, engineering, geography, international studies, liberal studies, psychology, and sociology.

I distributed faculty evaluation forms mandated by the university. In addition, an open-ended questionnaire was also used to assess information about course content, assignments, guest speakers, and videos. Students rated the course content on a scale ranging from 5 (strongly agree) to 1 (strongly disagree). The overall rating for course content was positive ($M = 4.91$, $SD = .28$). Moreover, a majority of the students stated that the assignments/activities were useful for learning and understanding the subject ($M = 4.88$, $SD = .32$).

On the open-ended evaluation form, many students stated that they really enjoyed taking the course and found the contents very interesting and informative. Examples of student comments include, "I have learned so much from taking this course. I am now more appreciative of other cultures. I will take this information and will use it for the rest of my life," and "Taking this course has opened my mind to cultural diversity that exists within the United States. I am now more aware and respectful of cultural differences. Whereas before, I would be more critical of different people's cultural customs, I now have a new found respect for their differences." "This class has been one of the most interesting classes that I have taken, I have learned a lot. I think this is a class everyone should take. It is so important now-a-days to be culturally open-minded."

Almost all the students (95%) indicated that they found the reading assignments interesting, informative, and educational. One student noted, "The readings significantly increased my understanding about other cultures and the way they live. I was so intrigued by some of them that I shared the information with my husband and we got into long discussions."

The students particularly enjoyed the videos. One student commented, "This class really increased my overall awareness and made me realize how ethnocentric I was. The videos were great and helped me in my understanding of the various cultures." Many students commented that the video, "Shadow of Hate," was particularly powerful and moving.

Many students stated that they acquired in-depth knowledge about a specific culture in working on the critical analysis group paper. A few students commented that working on a group project was slightly challenging because it was difficult to coordinate the different schedules.

Students wrote that they wanted more class discussions. Since the class was ethnically so diverse, they wished more students had shared their personal ideas and experiences. One student stated, "I wish some of the students from the minority ethnic groups shared their experiences with regard to discrimination and cultural adjustment with us." Also, some students indicated that they wished that the instructor had incorporated more guest speakers and videos in the course. Finally, a few students (all Euro-Americans) expressed the opinion that some of the views presented in the readings and videos seemed to be culturally-biased and that Euro-Americans were portrayed as bigots, racists, and exploiters. Despite this, all the students indicated that this should be a required course for Child Development and Family Studies majors and other pre-professionals planning to work in the field of Human Services.

## *CONCLUSION*

Education in the 21st century should be culturally sensitive, and constantly adapting to the changing needs of the students and an internationally diverse society. Undergraduate and graduate programs in family studies may find it necessary to introduce and accommodate courses on cultural and international families in their curriculum. Le Roux (2002) stressed that "effective education develops an understanding of others and their backgrounds, values, and traditions. It creates an intercultural awareness and sensitivity, and a realization of our interdependent local, regional and global existence" (p. 39).

Undergraduate students in family studies will be better served when their academic curriculum reflects the infusion of cultural diversity of international families in their courses. Although developing and teaching a course on international families maybe difficult, time consuming, and challenging for the instructor, the increased cultural awareness, knowledge, and personal growth of students taking the course is an excellent and indirect incentive and reward.

## REFERENCES

ABC Television Network. (1997, April 18). *The Hajj* [Television broadcast]. New York: ABC.

About, Inc. (2005). World atlas: Maps and geography of the world. Retrieved March 30, 2005, from http://geography.about.com/library/maps/blindex.htm

al Fārūqī & al Fārūqī, L. L. (1986). The cultural atlas of Islam. New York: Macmillan Reference USA.
American Psychological Association, Office of Program Consultation and Accreditation. (1996). Book 1: Guidelines and principles for accreditation of programs in professional psychology, and Book 2: Accreditation operating procedures. Washington, D.C.: Author.
Banks, J. A. (1995). Multicultural education and curriculum transformation. The Journal of Negro Education, 64, 390-400.
Banks, J. A. (2003). Teaching strategies for ethnic studies (7th ed.). Boston, MA: Allyn and Bacon.
Benokraitis, N. V. (2002). The changing ethnic profile of U.S. families in the twenty-first century. In N. V. Benokraitis (Ed.), Contemporary ethnic families in the United States (pp. 1-14). New Jersey: Prentice Hall.
Bosner, P. (Producer/Director). (1991). Race and ethnicity [Motion picture]. United States: Insight Media.
Carolan, M. T. & Mouton-Sanders, M. (2003). Islam. In J. J. Ponzetti (Ed.), International encyclopedia of marriage and family (pp. 956-960). New York: Macmillan Reference USA.
Central Intelligence Agency. (n.d.). The world factbook: Reference maps. Retrieved March 30, 2005, from http:www.cia.gov/cia/publications/factbook/docs/refmaps.html
Consulate General of India. (n.d.). Indian information: Land and the people. Retrieved September 22, 2003, from http://www.indianconsulate-sf.org
DeFrain, J. (2003). Family strengths. In J.J. Ponzetti (Ed.), International encyclopedia of marriage and family (pp. 637-641). New York: Macmillan Reference USA.
Ember, C. R. & Ember, M. (2002). Cultural anthropology (10th ed.). New Jersey: Prentice Hall.
Ghaffarian, S. (1987). The acculturation of Iranians in the United States. Journal of Social Psychology, 127, 565-57.
Haddad, Y. Y., Hains, B., & Findly, E. (1984). The Islamic impact. Syracuse, New York: Syracuse University Press.
Hill, R. (1973). Strengths of black families. New York: National Urban League.
Hourani, A. H. (1991). A history of the Arab peoples. Cambridge, Massachusetts: The Belknap Press of Harvard University.
Jackson, L. C. (1999). Ethnocultural resistance to multicultural training: Students and faculty. Cultural Diversity & Ethnic Minority Psychology, 5, 27-36.
Jalali, B. (1996). Iranian families. In M. McGoldrick, J. K. Pearce, & J. Giordano (Eds.), Ethnicity and family therapy (pp. 289-309). New York: The Guilford Press.
Karp, H. B. & Sammour, H. Y. (2000). Workforce diversity training programs & dealing with resistance to diversity. College Student Journal, 34, 451-458.
Labriola, T. (Producer/Director). (1993). Asian-American cultures in the United States: Dealing with diversity [Motion picture]. United States: Communication Services.
Learning Seed. (1998). Understanding our differences: Mexican and Americans [Motion picture]. United States: Learning Seed.

Lee, C. L. & Zane, N. W. (Eds.). (1998). *Handbook of Asian American psychology.* Thousand Oaks, California: Sage Publications.

Le Roux, J. (2002). Effective educators are culturally competent communicators. *Intercultural Education, 13*, 37-48.

Long, D. E. (1979). *The Hajj today.* Albany, New York: State University of New York Press.

Medora, N. P., Larson, J. H., Hortaçsu, H., & Dave, P. (2000). Perceived attitudes towards romanticism: A cross-cultural study of American, Asian-Indian, and Turkish young adults. *Journal of Comparative Family Studies, 33*, 155-178.

Medora, N. P. (2003). India. In J. J. Ponzetti (Ed.), *International encyclopedia of marriage and family* (pp. 876-883). New York: Macmillan Reference USA.

Moyer, J. (Producer/Director). (2002). *India and her people* [Motion picture]. United States: Smithsonian Institute.

Murphy, R. E. (1989). *Cultural & social anthropology: An overture* (3rd ed.). Englewood Cliffs, New Jersey: Prentice Hall.

Nanda, S. & Warms, R. L. (2002). *Cultural anthropology* (7th ed.). Belmont, California: Wadsworth/Thomson Learning.

Nasr, S. H. (1981). *Islamic life and thought.* Albany, New York: State University of New York Press.

Okihiro, G. Y. (1993). Victimization of Asians in America. *World and I, 8*, 396.

Organista, P. B., Chun, K. M., & Marin, G. (2000). Teaching an undergraduate course on ethnic diversity. *Teaching Psychology, 27*, 13-17.

Peters, F. E. (1994). *The Hajj: The Muslim pilgrimage to Mecca and the holy places.* Princeton, New Jersey: Princeton University Press.

Puente, A. E., Blanch, E., Candland, D. K., Denmark, F. L., Laman, C., Lutsky, N., Reid, P. T., & Schiavo, R. S. (1993). Toward a psychology of variance: Increasing the presence and understanding of ethnic minorities in psychology. In T. V. McGovern (Ed.), *Handbook for enhancing undergraduate education in psychology* (pp. 71-92). Washington, DC: American Psychological Association.

Riggs, M. (Producer/Director). (1991). *Black is . . . black ain't.* [Motion picture]. United States: California Newsreel.

Roy, K. & MacDermid, S. M. (2003). Families in society. In D. J. Bredehoft, & M. J. Walcheski (Eds.), *Family life education: Integrating theory and practice* (pp. 59-67). Minneapolis, MN: National Council on Family Relations.

Seltzer, R., Frazier, M., & Ricks, I. (1995). Multiculturalism, race, and education. *The Journal of Negro Education, 64*, 124-140.

Stanton, M. E. (1995). Patterns of kinship and residence. In B. B. Ingoldsby & S. Smith (Eds.), *Families in multicultural perspective* (pp. 97-116). New York: The Guilford Press.

Sudo, P. (1993). The faith and the followers. *Scholastic Update, 126*, 2-6.

Teaching Tolerance. (1995). *The shadow of hate: A history of intolerance in America* [Motion picture]. United States: Teaching Tolerance.

United States Census Bureau. (2000). *State and county quick facts: USA.* Retrieved September 22, 2003, from http://quickfacts.census.gov/qfd/states/06000.html

Zhang, S. (1995). Measuring shaming in an ethnic context. *British Journal of Criminology, 35*, 248-263.

# LIST OF VIDEOS USED IN THE INTERNATIONAL FAMILIES COURSE

Asian-American Cultures in the United States: Dealing with Diversity. (1993). Producer Director: Tony Labriola.
Insight Media Inc.
2162 Broadway
New York, NY 10024-0621
Phone: 1.800.233.9910 or 212.721.6316
Fax: 212.799.5309
E-mail: custserv@insight-media.com
Price: $149.00 Length: 25 minutes.

Black Is . . . Black Ain't. (1991). Producer/Director: Marlon T. Riggs.
California Newsreel
Order Department
P.O. Box 2284
South Burlington, VT 05497
Phone: 877.811.7495
Fax: 802.846.1850
E-mail: contact@newsreel.org
Price: $195.00 Length: 87 minutes.

The Hajj. (April 18, 1997). Aired on ABC's Nightline, (Television broadcast).
ABC News
P.O. Box 807
New Hudson, MI 48165
Phone: 1.800.505.6139
Fax: 602.870.4760
E-mail: helpdesk@datapakservices.com
Price: $99.95 Length: 20 minutes.

India and Her Peoples. (2002). Producer/Director: John Moyer.
Human Studies Film Archives
Smithsonian Institution Museum Support Center, MRC 534
4210 Silver Hill Rd.
Suitland, MD 20746
Phone: 301-238-1315
Fax: 301-238-2883

Race and Ethnicity. (1991). Producer/Director: Paul Bosner.
Insight Media Inc.
2162 Broadway
New York, NY 10024-0621
Phone: 1.800.233.9910 or 212.721.6316
Fax: 212.799.5309
E-mail: custserv@insight-media.com
Price: $139.00 Length: 25 minutes.

The Shadow of Hate: A History of Intolerance in America. (1995).
Teaching Tolerance
Order Department
400 Washington Ave.
Montgomery, Alabama 36104
Phone: 334.956.8200
Fax: 334.956.8486
Website: www.tolerance.org

Price: Free to Schools. Length: 40 minutes.
Understanding Our Differences: Mexicans and Americans. (1998).
Learning Seed
330 Telser Road
Lake Zurich, Illinois 60047
Phone: 1.800.634.4941
Fax: 1.800.998.0854
E-mail: learnseed@aol.com
Price: $89.00 Length: 23 minutes.

# An Integrative Approach to Teaching Family Resource Management

Jeanne M. Hilton
Karen Kopera-Frye

**ABSTRACT.** Family resource management is one of ten substance areas that are required for certification in family life education (National Council on Family Relations, 2005). Unfortunately, few discipline-specific resources are available for faculty assigned to teach the family resource management course. A rich tradition of theory and practice in the field has stalled, with little conceptual development since the 1980s to guide faculty teaching the course. In response, we offer a new conceptual framework for teaching family resource management that extends previous models by integrating management with other functions of the family. Specific course objectives, methods of evaluation, classroom activities, recommended materials, and teaching strategies are provided. *[Article copies available for a fee from The Haworth Document Delivery Service: 1-800-HAWORTH. E-mail address: <docdelivery@haworthpress.com> Website: <http://www.HaworthPress.com> © 2005 by The Haworth Press, Inc. All rights reserved.]*

**KEYWORDS.** Conceptual framework, family resource management, teaching

---

Jeanne M. Hilton and Karen Kopera-Frye are affiliated with the University of Nevada, Reno.

Address correspondence to: Dr. Jeanne M. Hilton, Department of Human Development and Family Studies, University of Nevada, Reno, NV 89557-0131 (E-mail: hilton@unr.edu).

## INTRODUCTION

The National Council on Family Relations (NCFR) recognizes the critical role of management in family life education and has included it as one of ten substance areas required for all Certified Family Life Educators (Bredehoft & Cassidy, 1995). Family resource management represents a distinct discipline within family studies that addresses;

> an understanding of the decisions individuals and families make about developing and allocating resources including time, money, material assets, energy, friends, neighbors, and space, to meet their goals (e.g., goal setting and decision making; development and allocation of resources; social environment influences; life cycle and family structure influences; consumer issues and decisions). (Bredehoft & Cassidy, 1995)

Unfortunately, management courses are being phased out of many academic programs, and the emphasis on teaching family resource management is disappearing in favor of courses and programs in consumer sciences and financial management. To complicate the situation further, there is only one family resource management text available for teaching (Goldsmith, 2004), and it offers little of the spirit of management that infuses the texts of previous leaders in the field.

Carol Vickers (1986) has identified four distinct eras in the history of development of family resource management that led to the state of the discipline today. The focus in each of these eras was:

- Health, sanitation, and the economics of household production from 1900 through the 1930s
- Household equipment, efficiency and task simplification in the 1940s and early 1950s
- Family processes, resource use, and decision making in the 1950s and 1960s
- The development of systems frameworks based on ecological theory in the 1970s to 1980s.

In the most recent era of conceptual development, the works of Deacon and Firebaugh (1975), Gross, Crandall and Knoll (1980), Paolucci, Hall and Axin (1977), and Nickell, Rice and Tucker (1976) have dominated the field, with models and texts that presented family resource management in an ecological context. The defining characteristics of these models were their universal emphasis on systems theory and their focus on management as a unique phenomenon that could be studied separately from the psychological and social functioning of the family. This approach promoted a family economics/management identity within the larger domain of the family sciences.

## THE NEED FOR A NEW APPROACH

The third edition (2004) of Goldsmith's *Resource Management for Individuals and Families* is the only family resource management text currently in print. Professionals trained in family economics and management are concerned that the Goldsmith text does not fully reflect the depth and richness of the discipline, nor does it reflect or support existing practice and scholarship. With fewer specialists in the field, fewer doctoral programs to train specialists to provide leadership, and only one marginal text to guide those teaching management, instructors assigned to teach the course are left with few resources to guide them. Consequently, there has been a trend toward using personal finance and consumer courses to satisfy the need to address the economic functioning of the family. While both financial and consumer skills are important to the family (and translate more directly into career options), the family literature documents the unique contribution of management skills in maintaining family well-being, and finance and consumer courses are no substitute for the conceptual foundation for other family courses that is provided by a well-conceived family resource management course.

Management models from the 1970s and 1980s created a solid identity for family resource management, by focusing on management processes in the context of families and their environments. In creating that identity, management was studied as a separate subsystem of the family. However, day-to-day management is embedded in all other areas of family functioning, and psychological and social functioning overlaps with management. Therefore, there is a need for updated models of management that integrate the economic, social and psychological domains of family life into a model of family resource management that explains how individual- and family-level choices maintain, enhance, or diminish various levels of well-being and quality of life for families and their communities. The following conceptual model and strategies for teaching family resource management course are offered as a first step in meeting this challenge.

## DESCRIPTION OF THE COURSE

The Gross et al. model (1980, Figure 1) was used as the foundation for the expanded conceptual framework (Figure 2) that has been used to teach a family resource management course for undergraduate students majoring in Human Development and Family Studies (HDFS). Students study management processes used by individuals and families in the contexts of their environmental resources and constraints, gender, ethnicity, social class, and family structure. The processes include needs assessment, identification of guiding values and principles, resource identification and allocation, decision making, communication, negotiation, conflict resolution, emotion regulation, feedback, information processing, goal setting, problem solving, planning, and implementing.

Eleven course objectives are used to assess student learning. By the conclusion of the course, students are expected to:

1. Recognize the contribution of management to individual and family well being over the life cycle.
2. Analyze the interdependent relationships between the family and other systems in the environment.
3. Apply management theory to individual and family decision making behavior, especially as it is related to the identification and allocation of resources.
4. Compare theories and models used to study family resource management and business management.
5. Examine similarities and differences in families' management of resources among sub-cultural groups and across socio-economic levels.
6. Examine how families provide support and share resources by studying interfamily resource exchange across family structures, ethnic groups, and generations.
7. Identify the incidence, causes, consequences, and stereotypes of family poverty.
8. Consider strategies for preventing and reducing poverty at the individual, family, and societal levels.
9. Examine welfare reform and reauthorization as a resource-related policy issue.
10. Apply the principles of effective management using personalized management activities.
11. Complete an in-depth analysis of a problem, using management concepts.

## FIGURE 1. Management Model (Gross, Crandall, & Knoll, 1980)

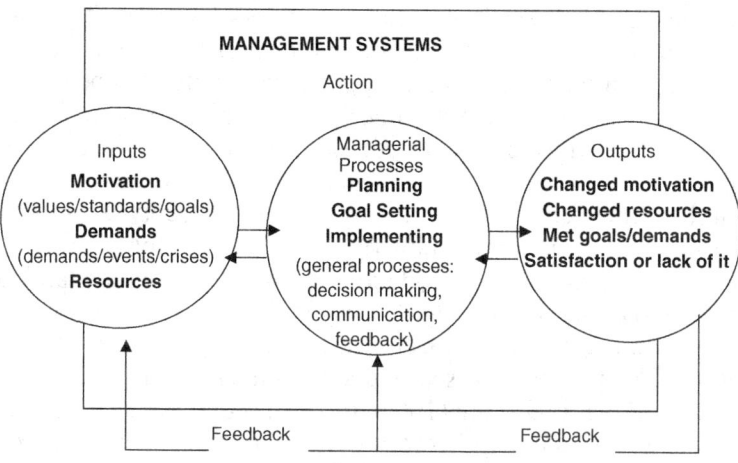

From Milstein, M. & Belasco, J. *Educational Administration and the Behavioral Sciences: A Systems Perspective.* Published by Allyn and Bacon, Boston, MA. Copyright © 1973 by Pearson Education. Adapted by permission of the publisher.

## FIGURE 2. New Management Model

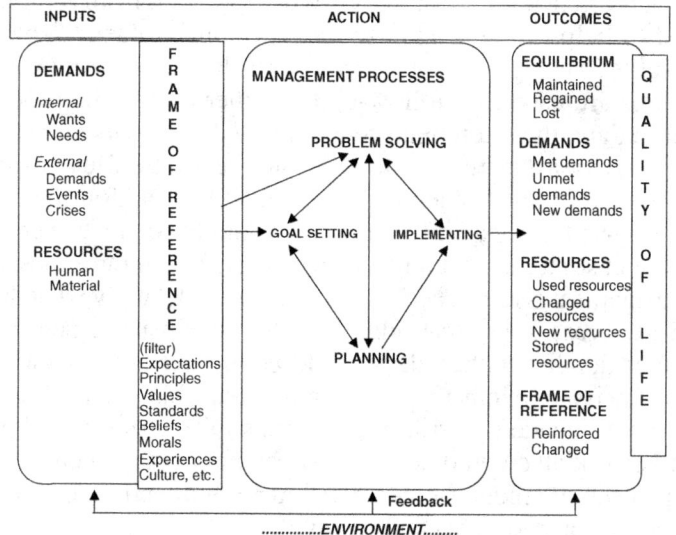

The first 10-11 weeks of the 15 week semester are dedicated to an in-depth examination of the various components of the management model, taking each section of the framework in order. The last five weeks constitute the applied portion of the course, where various topics are used to demonstrate how management principles can be used to address resource issues such as time management, stress management, and issues related to family structure, discrimination, social class, and resolving resource-based interpersonal conflicts. Students also examine research on interfamily resource exchange, the stereotypes, incidences, causes, and consequences of poverty, and welfare reform. Prerequisites for the course include the introductory human development and family courses, and either an introductory psychology or sociology course.

Course objectives are assessed in a variety of ways. Two exams (100 points each) are used to assess student's understanding of theory and concepts and the final exam (100 points) is used to assess their ability to apply theory and concepts to resource management issues. Students also engage in a case study developed for the course that requires them to identify an interpersonal problem, analyze how they might use what they have learned in class to resolve the problem, create an action plan, attempt to resolve the problem, and then evaluate the process and the outcome in a 5-page paper (see Table 1).

Students are also asked to participate in several independent and in-class activities that help them apply concepts and processes to real-life experiences. Two of the activities (adapted from Smith, 2000), are used to help students analyze their personal values (Table 2) and goals (Table 3) using concepts presented in class. Small group and class discussions are used as a follow-up to further clarify the processes of goal setting and the interconnectedness of values, goals and standards. A third activity asks students to evaluate the similarities, differences, and usefulness of third generation (Lakein, 1998) and fourth generation (Covey, 1989) time management models and to identify specific time management strategies that might help them with their three most difficult time management issues. Then students are asked to apply what they have learned to a case study that addresses the time management issues of dual-earner families. Other ideas would be to have students analyze the management issues of other types of families (e.g., blue-collar; dual-career; single parent; blended; at risk; grandparents raising grandchildren, etc.). The framework also could be used to design a management-related research project, or students could develop recommendations for prevention/intervention programs and policy.

## TABLE 1. Case Study in Problem Solving

Select a problem from your work or personal life that is frustrating to you and involves another person. Describe the problem in detail and then use your text, the principles outlined in class, and the following exercises to try to work through the problem. These exercises will help you to put into practice some of the concepts and skills you are trying to learn. After you have worked through the exercises, report your results in writing. Be sure to include information about all of the 7 steps below and use the concepts (and related terms) in your discussion, so I know that you can apply them. Your report should be typed, double-spaced and not more than 5 pages long. You will be graded on your ability to apply the concepts and principles to your situation and your ability to communicate this information in writing. Please address each of the following in your report:

1. Brainstorm the kinds of steps you might take to help resolve the problem. Which of these steps involve trying to change someone else's behavior? Which of the steps involve trying to change your own behavior? Evaluate what you can and cannot control in this situation.
2. Identify how you have behaved reactively to such problems in the past and explore how you could respond proactively to the problem this time.
3. Try to identify activities that are important but not urgent, that you know have been neglected in your life, and describe how paying attention to these activities might have prevented or minimized this problem (e.g., planning ahead, choosing your words carefully, investing time/energy in a relationship, or taking care of small problems before they get out of hand).
4. Analyze your scripting for conflict resolution. Is it competitive or cooperative? How does your scripting affect your interactions with other people? Can you identify the main source of your script (e.g., peers, parents, culture)?
5. After you have worked through the above exercises, try to develop a win/win solution to your problem. Put yourself in the other person's place, and write down what you think he/she wants. Then write down, from your own perspective, what results would constitute a win for you. What do you need from yourself and the other person to feel a sense of resolution? Are there areas of agreement between the two of you? Could you build on these?
6. Next, talk to the other person about the problem; listen carefully and try to understand the person's point of view (even if you don't agree with it), comparing what you are hearing with what you wrote down. How valid were your assumptions? Did you really understand the other person's perspective? What did you learn about listening with an open mind? Did your perspective on the problem change when you really understood the other person's point of view?
7. Now approach the other person and try to communicate and negotiate until you reach a point of agreement and a mutually beneficial win/win solution. Base your discussion on empathy and respect. First describe the other person's point of view as well or better than he or she can; then seek to have your perspective understood explaining it using the other person's frame of reference. Acknowledge areas of agreement and use your differences as stimuli for finding creative alternatives that promote win/win solutions. Start and end your conversation on a positive note, sandwiching the concerns in the middle.
8. Summarize your experience. Were you successful in resolving the problem? If not, what prevented you from finding a solution? Are you satisfied with the results? What did you learn about problem solving and conflict resolution from this experience?

## *The Conceptual Framework*

The framework used for the course contains several departures from Gross et al.'s (1980) model of management. In brief, their model identifies internal motivation (values, goals, and standards), external motivation (demand, events, and crises) and resources as inputs into the

## TABLE 2. Values Activity*

Part 1. Identify 10 of your top values and then write a clarifying statement for each. A list of some possible values is attached to help you. Please feel free to add to the list. What do you mean when you use the word for the value? For example, here are two of my personal values with clarifying statements to explain what the value means to me:

Value: TRANQUILITY

Clarifying statement:
Tranquility is inner peace and calm. It anchors me and gives me a sense of security. Tranquility allows me to live fully and to feel serene.

Value: UNCONDITIONAL LOVE

Clarifying statement:
Unconditional love has no strings attached, no matter what the circumstances may be. It is total acceptance of others as they are, the ability to forgive and let go, and a sincere desire for their growth and happiness, even when it is not in my own best interest.

---

### Examples of Values

| | | | | |
|---|---|---|---|---|
| Adventure | Enjoyment | Gracious living | Leadership | Prosperity |
| Authenticity | Excellence | Gratitude | Learning/ | Purposefulness |
| Balance | Faith | Growth | education | Quality |
| Beauty | Family | Health | Loyalty | Respect |
| Being centered | Financial | Honesty | Love | Responsibility |
| Career | security | Humility | Optimism | Spirituality |
| Companionship | Fitness | Humor | Patience | Teamwork |
| Comfort | Freedom | Innovation | Persistence | Tranquility |
| Courage | Generosity | Integrity | Playfulness | Unconditional love |
| Creativity | Good attitude | Joyfulness | Pleasure | Vitality |
| | | | Professionalism | Wisdom |

---

Part 2. Now write your top four values in the boxes below . . . we will use this part of the assignment in the class discussion.

| | |
|---|---|
| Value 1 | Value 2 |
| Value 3 | Value 4 |

*(Adapted from Smith, 2000)

## TABLE 3. Goals Activity*

Part 1. Identify your roles. A role describes who you are and what you do. Another way to think of it is that our roles are the different "hats" that we wear as we go about our daily lives . . . family member, worker, friend, manager, volunteer, etc. Starting by identifying our roles is helpful in setting goals, because it gives us a framework for thinking through what we want to accomplish in each area of our lives.

Identify your roles (no more than 5 categories for the assignment). Then identify the key people you associate with in each role and write a clarifying statement for each of the roles you listed. Imagine what the key people would say about you if you were doing a completely outstanding job in this role. For example, the key people involved with my teaching are students, other faculty, and the dean. What do these people expect from me? Here is the clarifying statement in response to my question:

ROLE: Teacher
KEY PEOPLE: Students, Faculty, Dean
CLARIFYING STATEMENT: "I lead and stay up-to-date. I make learning fun. I give students time to process what they are learning. I advise with patience and concern. I help the teaching program improve and run smoothly."

Part 2. Now, consider what matters most to you. Use the following questions to help you think about your life's purpose. As you answer these questions and think about your key roles, your goals will begin to emerge. This is also useful if you want to write a personal mission statement.

- If you were to do one thing in your professional life that would have the most positive impact on your life, what would that one thing be?
- If you were to do one thing in your personal life that would have the most positive impact on your life, what would that one thing be?
- List all the things you would like to have in your lifetime (e.g., new home, children, travel to Europe, etc.).
- List all the things you would like to do in your lifetime (e.g., travel to every continent, get a graduate degree, see the Northern Lights, etc.).
- What kind of a person do you want to be (e.g., fun-loving, ambitious, responsible, compassionate, etc.)?
- What have been some of your greatest moments of happiness and fulfillment?
- What activities do you most enjoy and find fulfilling?
- What talents and/or abilities do you have or want to have?
- How can you best contribute to the world?
- If your life were cut short by an accident or illness, what would you want most to have done with the time you had? What would you regret?

Part 3. Write down your goals. Set one goal for each of the 5 most important roles that you identified in the first step. Each goal should be specific, measurable, action oriented, realistic, and you should be able to accomplish it within the next year.

*(Adapted from Smith, 2000)

managerial sub-system. Motivations are matched with resources in the managerial portion of the model, using specific managerial processes (goal setting, planning and implementation of plans). Decision-making, communication and feedback are viewed as general processes that are embedded in the more specific functions of the managerial processes. The outcome of management is viewed as satisfaction or lack of satisfaction with choices that were made, as well as the impact on larger systems in the environment.

In the revised model, two types of environments influence inputs into the action or managerial portion of the model. The internal environment constitutes the motivations (wants and needs) and perceptions (frame of reference) of individual family members and the family system; the external environment includes other systems and conditions that shape demands placed upon individuals and families. The action component of the model (processes of management), includes setting individual and family level goals, creating plans to carry out the goals, implementing the plans and problem solving as needed, to keep the other management processes moving forward. Decision making, communication, and feedback are general processes embedded in all aspects of management. The outcome of management has been redefined to better reflect the contextual nature and impact of management on individuals, family systems and their environments.

## Inputs into the Management System

*Internal and External Sources of Motivation.* Wants and needs are the foundation of human motivation. These motivators arise internally within the individual and the family, and externally through demands made on the family from other systems. Because human, material, and financial resources are limited, choices have to be made among a multitude of options. Basic needs must be satisfied for normal functioning (although the timing for satisfying the need may be an option), whereas wants are optional. Norwood (1999) provides a model that builds on Maslow's (1971) hierarchy of needs to describe the types of information that individuals seek as they attempt to meet their different needs. Both individuals and families seek coping information to satisfy their physiological needs, helping information to meet the need for safety, enlightening information to meet the need for belonging, empowering information to meet the need for esteem, and edifying information to meet the need for self-actualization and self-transcendence.

*Spirituality as a Basic Need.* Spirituality has largely been ignored in both family resource management and in other family sciences. When spirituality is addressed at all, it is usually framed in the context of religious attendance. However, spirituality has been recognized as a basic human need (Tischler, Biberman, & McKeage, 2002). Religious people may or may not be spiritual. Spiritual people may or may not be religious.

Spirituality has been described as the basic feeling of being connected to one's complete self, others, and the entire universe (Mitroff & Denton, 1999, p. 83). Others have defined spirituality as our inner consciousness (Guillory, 2000, p. 33), or as an inner search for meaning or fulfillment (Graber, 2001, p. 40). In his later model, Maslow (1971) proposed that self-transcendence (a form of spirituality) is the highest order human need (above self-actualization), and that lower level needs have to be met before self-transcendence can occur.

However, there is little empirical evidence that human needs operate hierarchically as Maslow has proposed (Dintelman, 2002). For example, in third world countries around the world, people who cannot reliably meet the most basic needs for food, shelter, and safety find ways to be loving, generous, joyful, and creative, in spite of their hardships. In addition, we have all observed that in the midst of a crisis or at the end of life, when all is slipping away, many individuals find a spiritual connection that brings closure, comfort and peace.

All cultures across time have embraced some form of spiritual expression. Therefore, it appears that spirituality is a universal need that we all have, and the search for meaning is essential to our physical and psychological survival. In this sense, the role of spirituality in constructing meaning in life, in making gut-wrenching decisions, in solving ethical problems, and in values formation takes on critical importance in understanding how families thrive and grow. Basing such choices on larger meaning, a connection to the whole, and searching for guiding principles appears to be a more powerful management strategy, than relying on individual or family values. Unlike universally sound principles, values are not necessarily morally sound or ethical. Gross et al. (1980) considered values, goals, and standards to be internal motivations that prompt managerial efforts. In the current framework, the search for meaning (spirituality) is considered to be a basic human need, and values and standards are part of the frame of reference or filter that influences how individuals and families perceive their wants and needs.

*The Frame of Reference.* Each family member brings his or her own perceptions of reality to the table when family members interact. In earlier management models, little attention was paid to the internal environment that shapes family members' perceptions of reality, the conflicts that arise when perceptions of reality clash and the muddled soup of emotions that are at play when family members attempt to meet the multiple and often conflicting needs of themselves and others in their social and economic environments. This internal environment is conceptualized as a "frame of reference," but other terms such as a perception of reality or the internal filter could be used. The frame of reference or internal filter is shaped, in part, by culture, cohort, gender, and ethnicity and includes individual and family values, standards, principles, beliefs, emotional tone and so on. No two family members share exactly the same frame of reference. Therefore, a large part of family resource management involves making family level choices within these individualized (and often conflicting) perceptions of reality.

Humans, in general as well as within the family, are prone to assume that their view of reality IS reality and that it is shared by others. An effective strategy for teaching this concept is to carry a bottle of water to class and use the labeling on the bottle to illustrate that each of us has a different view of the world that we live in. The class sees the front of the bottle and the instructor sees the back. Until the bottle is turned or someone tries to look at the other side of the bottle, each individual will see only part of the picture. Neither view is reality. Both views are reality. Taken *together*, these views are closer to reality than any one view by itself. Differences are not wrong or bad . . . they are just different. There is something to be learned by listening to other points of view. This fundamental assumption about reality is a powerful management tool that is truly accepting of diversity in all of its forms, and it is a key concept for understanding the dynamics of family functioning.

## *Management Processes*

Communication, decision making and feedback. Management involves three general processes (communication, decision making and feedback) that are embedded in the specific processes of management: goal setting, problem solving, planning and implementing. Communication involves giving and getting information, decision making involves making choices among options, and feedback involves giving and getting cues to regulate stability and change in the system. All three are used as the family and its members attempt to make choices among options available to them, in the context of limited resources.

*Goal setting, planning and implementing* are three processes specific to the action or management portion of the model. Goal setting involves deciding which wants and needs the individual or family will attempt to satisfy within a specified time frame. Three processes are used in goal setting: (1) *Selection* is used to choose those options (goals) that will or will not be pursued, given available resources, (2) *Optimization* involves setting growth- or gain-related goals to get the best payoff from the use of limited resources, and (3) *Compensation* involves using alternative goal strategies and substitutions to maintain functioning and minimize losses (Baltes, Baltes, Freund, & Lang, 1999; Baltes & Smith, 2003; Freund & Baltes, 1998). Present circumstances, available resources, and each family member's frame of reference helps shape the specific criteria (standards) for each goal.

Planning and implementing are used to carry out the goals that individuals and families have set. Planning involves creating a sequence of steps or a mental creation of future actions that will result in goal attainment. Implementing involves putting the plan into action, checking to see that progress is being made, and making adjustments, when necessary.

*Problem Solving.* Problem solving involves removing obstacles that block goal attainment. The work of the major theorists in the 1970s and 1980s (Deacon & Firebaugh, 1975; Gross et al., 1980; Paolucci et al., 1977; Rice & Tucker, 1986) paid little attention to problem solving even though it is a critical component of management. Every process within the action component of management is knocked off course when unanticipated problems surface. Goals are blocked, plans have to be revised and renegotiated, and/or implementation of plans is interrupted until each presenting problem is somehow resolved. The problems that surface can range in scope from nuisances to crises, and the processes and strategies used to resolve problems and keep management processes on track are of central concern to those working with families.

Because we live in a world that is governed by many different views of what is real, appropriate, right, and fair, a large part of individual and family problem solving involves negotiating solutions, managing conflict and regulating emotional expression. Skills and strategies for managing emotion and conflict need to be fostered and learned in the classroom, and modalities for teaching these skills need to be developed and modeled for future family life educators.

There is an entire body of literature on conflict management in interpersonal and family relationships that can be adapted and used in family resource management courses. In the contexts of both the communication and problem solving processes, students are taught strategies to use when the other person is upset, what to do when the student is upset, and what to do when both parties are upset (regulate conflict) or neither is upset (invest in building the relationship). Some of the strategies include listening with empathy, owning a problem, distancing or time-out when discussions get too heated, and setting limits.

Laurel Mellin's (1997) book, *The Solution*, is based on a program sponsored by the U. C. San Francisco medical school. The text is an excellent resource for teaching students about emotion regulation. Formal training for faculty is available through self-study and by certified and licensed health care professionals. Students learn about the cascade (i.e., progressive levels) of emotion (anger, sadness, fear, regret, and acceptance) and how to work through the levels on their own or with help when necessary. They learn to identify and label their feelings, the unmet needs underlying their feelings, and to assess whether they can meet their needs on their own, or whether they need some type of support. They also learn to identify their expectations for themselves and whether or not they are reasonable, to reframe their expectations to be reasonable (not too high or too low), to reframe their thoughts to be powerful and positive, and to distinguish between unavoidable emotional pain and the unnecessary pain that they bring upon themselves. They learn that unavoidable pain will pass and that they have control over avoidable pain.

Nurturing and setting limits are considered to be the basic skills of competent parents. Those who are raised in healthy families have these needs met throughout childhood and learn self-regulation over time. Those who are raised in less favorable environments have to learn these basic skills in adulthood. The skills-based approach (in contrast to a problem-focused or deficit approach) is empowering for students, and for family life professionals and their clients. Students who do not have these skills need to learn them before they take on professional roles working with vulnerable families. As professionals, they can use these skills to work through problems with clients, but what is more important is that they can teach these skills to their clients so that they eventually have the necessary tools to handle their own problems.

The solutions approach is demonstrated in class with two student volunteers. One is asked to think of a distressing situation to work on, one that would not be too personal to discuss in front of the class. The second student is asked to serve as scribe by writing all responses under the appropriate headings on the board. The teacher asks the student questions from the solutions process, probing where necessary, and the scribe writes the student's responses on the board under each question. The class watches as the student processes the problem and comes up with strategies for solving it. Changes in the processing of emotion are also noted (e.g., the student has gained insight, is no longer angry, etc.). The comments on the board give students a visual map of how the process works. After the activity is finished, students are invited to discuss their observations and ask the student volunteer questions about his/her experience with the process.

*Family-level problem solving* is also addressed in the course. This is a relatively new field of study that was created by social and behavioral scientists about thirty years ago.

Vuchinich (1999) has written an excellent book on this topic, and offers definitions for both family problems and family problem solving.

> *Family problems* are conditions that block the attainment of individual or family goals. These conditions may include behaviors, rules, expectations, attitudes, relationships, social structures, action patterns, or circumstances external to the family. (p. 11)

> *Family problem solving* is the removal of conditions that block the attainment of family-based goal. (p. 12)

Vuchinich (1999) traces the origins of current thinking about family problem solving and uses theory to address the social nature of problems, the social construction of family problems, solutions to the family's social constructions, and the phases and sequences involved in family problem solving. He also offers chapters devoted to application of family problem solving in troubled family systems, as well as strategies for teaching family problem solving skills in prevention programs and parenting education. Faculty teaching lower division courses may want to use this text as a resource in developing course materials. Those teaching upper division or graduate courses may want to consider using the book as a required text.

## *Management Outcomes*

Management outcomes have been minimally addressed in most texts, past and present. For the most part, outputs of the managerial system have been categorized as met demands, used resources and satisfaction or lack of it, or as the degree of success in meeting goals. Gross et al.

(1980) also briefly address the broader impact of management activities on the psycho-social, physical, and political-economic systems, and Rice and Tucker (1986) present a thorough discussion of lifestyle and quality of life as endpoints of management. Surprisingly, Deacon and Firebaugh (1975) have little to say about the effects of family resource management on other systems in their chapter on outcomes, and Goldsmith (2004) ignores the topic altogether.

The adapted framework addresses changes in demands, resources, and the frame of reference that occur as a result of managerial efforts. Changes in the equilibrium of the family system have been added as an additional key outcome. Much of what management entails concerns families' efforts to maintain the status quo, deliberately introduce desired changes into the family system, and/or adapt to undesired or unanticipated demands on the system. Therefore, any assessment of outcome should address whether specific management efforts have helped the family system to maintain, regain, or lose its equilibrium.

Flach (1999) offers an interesting perspective on equilibrium as an outcome. He proposes that in the normal course of individual and family development, and with externally imposed crises, bifurcation points occur. Flach (1999) defines a bifurcation as a time of extreme change when a system becomes destabilized. When major change occurs, individuals and families typically "fall apart" and then regroup. Flach believes that disorganization is normal, and sometimes even necessary, for adaptation to take place. Families deconstruct and then reconstruct their realities.

Developmental milestones and crises create bifurcation points across the life course. Developmental milestones can occur at both the individual and family levels, such as when individuals transition from one life stage to the next (childhood to adolescence) or at the family level, when a family system adds or loses a member through birth, marriage, divorce, remarriage, children leaving home, or death. At each of these transition points, disequilibrium occurs and the system must reorganize and reintegrate. Non-normative events and crises also disrupt the family system and create the need to reintegrate. In either case, Flach (1999) suggests that reintegration occurs at four levels: resilient reintegration, homeostatic reintegration, maladaptive reintegration, and dysfunctional reintegration. In other words, the family's functioning in response to the management of developmental transitions and crises can improve, stay the same or deteriorate.

Other outcomes traditionally identified within our field tend to focus on the family's satisfaction or lack of satisfaction with goal attainment (getting what the family wants and needs). Although Rice and Tucker (1985) is an exception, less attention has been paid to the ultimate outcome of management: its impact on the quality of life for everyone–individuals, families, and their communities. In a truly ecological management model, the need for respecting the principle of maintaining balance among the major domains of human functioning and across ecological systems needs to be stressed, and the quality of life of individuals, the family, and the community needs to be highlighted as the ultimate end point of the family's managerial efforts.

## CONCLUSION

The conceptual framework that has been described builds on a rich tradition of theory and practice in the field of family resource management, and extends previous work by adding conceptual material and integrating management and the psychological and social functioning of the family. The model illustrates the complexity of management processes, the interdependence of management with other functions of the family, and the ecological impact of the family's day-to-day choices. It also provides structure for teaching the course and gives students a framework for analyzing when, where, and how management processes and family functioning might be thriving or failing. The interdependence among family members, the family system, and its environments are stressed and various assignments and activities help students to explore their own management skills and strategies and apply management concepts to different types of families. The family resource management course offers students a unique opportunity to integrate the various levels of family functioning and to learn specific information and practical skills that will be invaluable to them in other family courses, and as they move into their roles as human service professionals and family life.

## REFERENCES

Baltes, P. B., Baltes, M. M., Freund, A. M. & Lang, F. R. (1999). *The measure of selective optimization with compensation (SOC) by self-report (Technical Report 1999)*. Berlin, Germany: Max Planck Institute for Human Development.

Baltes, P. B. & Smith, J. (2003). New frontiers in the future of aging: From successful aging of the young old to the dilemmas of the fourth age. *Journals of Gerontology: Behavioral Sciences, 49*, 123-135.

Bredehoft, D. & Cassidy, D. (Eds). (1995). College and university curriculum guidelines in Family Life Education. Minnesota: National Council on Family Relations. Retrieved 6-22-05 from http://www.ncfr.org/pdf/FLE_Substance_Areas.pdf

Covey, S. R. (1989). *The 7 habits of highly effective people.* New York, NY: Fireside Publishers.

Deacon, R. & Firebaugh, F. (1975). *Home management context and concepts.* Boston, MA: Houghton, Mifflin & Co.

Dintelman, B. (2002). *Maslow's hierarchy of needs.* Retrieved March 2002 from http://www.iejs.com/Management/maslows_hierarchy_of_needs.htm

Flach, F. (1999). *Resilience: The power to bounce back when the going gets tough!* New York, NY: Hatherleigh Press.

Freund A. M. & Baltes, P. B. (1998). Selection, optimization, and compensation as strategies of life management: Correlations with subjective indicators of successful aging. *Psychology and Aging, 13,* 531-543.

Graber, D. R. (2001). Spirituality and healthcare organizations. *Journal of Healthcare Management, 46,* 39-50.

Goldsmith, E. B. (2004). *Resource management for individuals and families* (3rd ed.). Belmont, CA: Wadsworth/Thompson Learning.

Gross, I. H., Crandall, E. W. & Knoll, M. M. (1980). *Management for modern families* (4th ed.). Indianapolis, IN: Prentice Hall.

Guillory, W. A. (2000). *The living organization: Spirituality in the workplace.* Salt Lake City, UT: Innovations International, Inc.

Hilton, J. M. (2004). *Family resource management: Revitalization for the 21st century.* Keynote presentation delivered at the 45th annual conference of the Western Family Economics Association, Honolulu, HI.

Lakein, A. (1998). *How to get control of your time and your life.* New York, NY: Penguin Group.

Maslow, A. (1971). *The farther reaches of human nature.* New York: The Viking Press.

Mellin, L. (1997). *The solution.* New York, NY: Harper/Collins.

Mitroff, I. I. & Denton, E. A. (1999). *A spiritual audit of corporate America.* San Francisco, CA: Jossey-Bass, Publishers.

Nickell, P., Rice, A. S., & Tucker, S. M. (1976). *Management in family living.* New York, NY: John Wiley & Co.

Norwood, G. (1999). *Maslow's hierarchy of needs: The truth vectors (Part 1).* Retrieved May 2002, from http://www.deepermind.com/20maslow.htm

Paolucci, B., Hall, O. A., & Axinn, N. W. (1977). *Family decision making: An ecosystems approach.* New York: John Wiley & Co.

Rice, A. S. & Tucker, S. M. (1986). *Family life management* (6th ed.). New York, NY: Macmillan.

Smith, H. W. (2000). *What matters most: The power of living your values.* New York: Fireside Division of Simon & Schuster.

Tischler, L., Biberman, J. & McKeage, R. (2002). Linking emotional intelligence, spirituality and workplace performance: Definitions, models and ideas for research. *Journal of Managerial Psychology, 17,* 203-218.

Vickers, C. (1984). *Themes in home economics and their impact on families, 1909-1984.* Washington, DC: American Home Economics Association.

Vuchinich, S. (1999). *Problem solving in families: Research and practice.* Thousand Oaks, CA: Sage.

# *TEACHING TECHNIQUES IN FAMILY STUDIES*

# Creating Families: A Teaching Technique for Clinical Training Through Role-Playing

Scott Browning
Jeanne S. Collins
Bryan Nelson

**ABSTRACT.** This article examines an alternative marriage and family teaching method that provides students with a realistic clinical experience and increases their empathic understanding of family diversity. When the instructor incorporates a highly structured role-play protocol into the syllabus, students learn to create realistic family scenarios, without falling prey to the two main traps of role-play: the ill-prepared example that does not represent real cases; and the ethical problem in which students select characters too similar to themselves. *[Article copies available for a fee from The Haworth Document Delivery Service: 1-800-HAWORTH. E-mail address: <docdelivery@haworthpress.com> Website: <http://www.HaworthPress.com> © 2005 by The Haworth Press, Inc. All rights reserved.]*

**KEYWORDS.** Classroom simulation, clinical training, role-play, teaching family diversity

---

Scott Browning, Jeanne S. Collins, and Bryan Nelson are all affiliated with Chestnut Hill College.

Address correspondence to: Scott Browning, Professor, Department of Psychology, Chestnut Hill College, 9601 Germantown Avenue, Philadelphia, PA 19118 (E-mail: scobrown@chc.edu).

© 2005 by The Haworth Press, Inc. All rights reserved.
doi:10.1300/J002v38n04_01

## INTRODUCTION

Teaching the prospective therapist about "the family" requires training methods that provide the student with both a theoretical base and a practical application. However, in marital and family therapy, implementing experiential instruction that provides insight into family processes has become a difficult challenge. Because practical and ethical concerns have restricted the instructional use of real families and actual therapy sessions, role-playing has become an increasingly important instructional technique. This paper describes a novel approach to role-playing, Creating Families, which addresses some of the shortcomings traditionally associated with role-playing methods.

## EXPERIENTIAL CLINICAL TRAINING TECHNIQUES

Experiential activities provide students with the ability to supplement didactic training with observation and practice of therapeutic skills. Several educators have reported that experiential teaching exercises can effectively expand students' frame of reference. Kim and Lyons (2003), for example, have described experiential activities, including games, as constructive strategies for instilling and improving multicultural competency, skills, awareness, and knowledge in counselor trainees. Helmeke and Prouty (2001) developed an experiential exercise to help marriage and family therapists-in-training cultivate their therapeutic skills, in which students playing clients spoke a language unfamiliar to the therapists, who had to try to understand the client in other ways. They assert that such experiential exercises can increase empathy and sensitivity to others' experiences, and help students better understand their preconceptions about others.

Yalom (2002) contends that observing therapy in practice is the best method for examining the clinical process and teaching skills to students. Although some training centers still offer observational opportunities for students, this type of experiential training has become less prevalent due to legal, ethical and practical concerns. In talking with students who have participated in the role-play process, one student reported that after spending time in character, she began to experience almost spontaneously her character's defenses, feelings, and responses to a given situation (Collins, 2004; Lindblad-Goldberg, personal communication, 2002). Consequently, role-play has supplemented the previous practice of observing videotaped session of actual therapy.

## BENEFITS AND CAVEATS OF ROLE-PLAY TEACHING EXERCISES

Role-play, in which a student assumes the character traits of a hypothetical person who will be treated by a student-therapist, is a useful and unique experiential method for teaching students clinical skills (Martin-Smith, 1995). Unlike lectures or discussions of required readings, role-play enables students to observe therapy without the associated risks to real clients. Role-play is different from the use of standardized patients, which is common for therapist training in Europe (VanderGraf, personal communication, 1998), but has remained an important component of medical education in the United States. While standardized patients adhere strictly to a "script" of behaviors and responses, role-play involves the creation of an individual character with a specific history, life circumstance, and personality.

Despite the benefits of role-play, however, there is the possibility that students may divulge personal or emotionally charged material during a role-play situation, requiring instructors to monitor it closely and apply restrictions when necessary. The American Psychological Association (2002) Ethical Principles of Psychologists and Code of Conduct and the American Association of Marriage and Family Therapists (2004) ethics code both stipulate that faculty members should not require students to disclose personal information in course-related activities. However, the ethical codes do allow for student disclosure when the course material clearly stipulates this requirement in advance.

Levitov, Fall and Jennings (1999) sidestepped some ethical and practical concerns of role-play by using trained student actors as clients instead of fellow classmates. They cautioned that student integration of confidential personal information into a client role-play, combined with the difficulty of determining what type of material to reveal, may lead to inappropriate personal disclosures. This may include breaches of confidentiality, and professional boundary issues that may lead to jeopardizing student relationships with faculty.

In a different approach to ethical concerns, Rabinowitz (1997) took on the client's role himself, while his students played the counselor's role. He asserted that students benefited from increased understanding of abstract concepts such as transference and the challenge of trying techniques they had read about or seen demonstrated. They also experienced surprise at the realism of the role-play as well as investment in the relationship with the client.

A significant drawback of the Levitov et al. (1999) and Rabinowitz (1997) models is that therapists-in-training never play the client's role, making it difficult to develop the same degree of empathy as students who take on the role of client. Empathy is a vitally important aspect of both experiential learning and good therapy (Bohart & Greenberg, 1997). Furr and Carroll (2003), for example, reported that students in a master's counseling program repeatedly emphasized the value of assuming the client's role. They noted that the opportunity to take on the role of both client and counselor contributed greatly to the students' development as counselors.

An important way to increase empathy for a role-played character is by giving the character true depth. Shepard (2002) addressed the need to develop empathy and sensitivity for the interpersonal dynamics in the client-therapist relationship, and raised some of the ethical concerns of role-playing techniques. By employing a "screenwriting" protocol in which he helped students create believable, realistic, characters with depth, the students learned to act out their developed character and experience "being on the other side" (p. 148).

## APPLICATION OF ROLE-PLAY TO FAMILY THERAPY

The general benefits of role-play as a learning technique apply strongly and specifically to teaching family therapy, especially for topics for which there are no other obvious methods for increasing student understanding. The ability for multiple characters to "work off" one another frequently contributes to more realistic results in a significant manner. Role-playing a particular family type enables the student to recognize the importance of issues common to structurally similar families, such as feeling "stuck in the middle" within a stepfamily. Role-play allows students to develop and expand their understanding of family emotions, dilemmas, dynamics, and diversity in ways not possible through didactic instruction alone. A student who has directly experienced the dilemmas that are common in stepfamily life, or the predictable developmental sequences that family members experience following the adoption of a child, is likely to be more actively engaged in a traditional classroom setting.

Notwithstanding these benefits, few family therapy role-play teaching techniques appear to satisfy both ethical and experiential requirements. Banyard and Fernald (2002), for example, developed a classroom-based method for family therapy role-play. However, their protocol is time-limited, provides few guidelines for character development, and may not prepare students adequately to differentiate between projected or personal material, or protect them from disclosing personal information. While Shepard's (2002) screenwriting protocol addresses the need for both safe and emotionally valuable role-play, his techniques are limited to individual therapy situations.

## AN ALTERNATIVE: THE "CREATING FAMILY" PROTOCOL

The "Creating Family" role-play protocol provides the experiential benefits of role-playing in a family therapy situation, while also protecting the student. Designed at Chestnut Hill College in Philadelphia, the protocol has been refined and informally validated over 10 years with dozens of students and faculty members at selected graduate programs (The Wright Institute, Colorado State University, Massachusetts School of Professional Psychology, The University of British Columbia). Some of these formed "created families" were also used by the training faculty of the Stepfamily Association of America to exhibit clinical techniques to a professional audience.

The following 14 steps outline a procedure for creating realistic families while attending to the ethical concerns of engaging students in role-play. The first nine steps deal directly with the creation of the "family," while the last five steps address using this tool as a teaching model.

### Step 1: Build the Family Creation Process into Your Course Outline

The protocol described here may be used either to create a single "clinical family" for each member of the class to treat, or in larger classes, several "families" may be created simultaneously. Although a single family may include up to five students, the process seems to work best if the family size is limited to three or four. The instructor(s) can move between groups, spending enough time with each to provide adequate guidance.

### Step 2: Determine the Type of Family to Be Created

Examples of family types we have created include: (a) stepfamilies, (b) divorced families, (c) gay and lesbian families, (d) single-parent families, (e) multi-racial stepfamilies, (f) multi-racial first-marriage families, (g) families with an addicted member, (h) families with "special needs," (i) families with a troubled adolescent, (j) foster-care families, and (k) three-generation families in a single residence. The age, gender, or race of the students is important in selecting family types and compositions. Although students can role-play someone younger, older, or of the opposite gender, they must be convincing in the role. Students who wish to play a particular role must be asked if they have the ability to perceive the character realistically.

## Step 3: Build the Dynamics of the Family

The formation of the family is a process that takes into account both physical appearance and student interests. The students determine who might be married or committed to whom and whether a particular student can effectively play, for example, a child connected to a given couple. Once the families have been created, the instructor sends student family units to separate rooms to discuss and build family dynamics. Several rules are implicit to this process, beginning with the caveat that anyone who finds a role personally too difficult to assume should request a change, without the need to specify a reason.

It is important that the instructor coaches the family in character and family creation and solicits opinions from others to assure input from a variety of participants. If the created family does not seem realistic, the instructor asks, "Would this family actually be seeking therapy?" The instructor also stipulates that when the students build the family, family secrets should be kept secret; in other words, anything heard by everyone involved cannot remain a secret. Students should be told that they should create secrets only while meeting in a subsystem during subsequent protocol steps (see Step 6).

## Step 4: Character Profile Development

Although the "family" develops initial details about its roles and structure, a process that should take about 2 hours of class time, each member of the created family should independently develop his or her character more fully outside the classroom. Students also should read several self-selected articles on clinical characteristics of their family's particular subtype, such as life in stepfamilies or foster care families. This research should not be exhaustive because remaining questions about clinical aspects will fuel the student's need to read more.

*Writing the character sketch.* Next, the students should write a character sketch, including some history, personal traits, current living situation, personal relationships, and presenting problems. Students should be encouraged to ask basic questions about the character and establish a clear rationale for the character's concerns and life situation. They should give names to the character and to the people in the character's life. Students should avoid choosing a character's profession beyond their own level of knowledge.

Besides planning the practical details of the characters' lives, students also should carefully construct coherent psychological profiles. For example, they should think about how a particular person typically experiences close relationships, relationships with authority figures, and which emotions present difficulties for this person. In addition, they should consider: (a) how the person defends against unpleasant emotions or stressful situations, (b) situations the person experiences as particularly stressful, (c) whether the person expresses emotions directly or indirectly, (d) the person's goals or aspirations, and (e) situations or emotions that typically evoke conflict for this person.

The goal is to create a specific, realistic person, not simply a diagnostic protocol. Although many students think in terms of symptoms and diagnosis, it is not necessary for the character to qualify clearly for a formal DSM-IV diagnosis. In fact, the role-play character is often more complex and interesting if students build the character with an emphasis on history. Therefore, students should create a character "from the ground up," rather than using a top-down approach that begins with a diagnosis and proceeds to simply "filling in the blanks." Although the protocol may be shifted toward an emphasis on disorder diagnosis in a course on psychopathology, students may need assistance in building their character.

As students construct this psychological profile, they should avoid creating a character too much like themselves or someone they know. Instead, they should strive to create a realistic composite character by incorporating some of their own and acquaintances' characteristics and attributes. It may seem easy and useful to base the character completely on an acquaintance (or a client), but this should be discouraged. To gain the most from this process, students must experience the actual *construction* of a character, rather than relying on their own history or the perceived life of someone they know. Instructors should remind students that because aspects of character will be discussed in class during interactions with the student-therapist, they should reduce their personal level of vulnerability by excluding many of their own traits.

*Profile development caveats.* Students should be encouraged to focus on the character rather than the acting. The purpose is to help students gain an understanding of human experience separate from their own, and to provide useful "clients" for clinical training. Students should experience the character role and form an overall picture, not attempt to turn the exercise into a method acting performance that distracts from the experiential goal of role-play.

Students should not create a character and then take an outside perspective of the character they have created. In other words, while "in character" the student should not try to explain their own character's motivation, any more than any person can explain their motivation in real life. For example, if the student creates a character that suffered a trauma, the "character" should not hint around the topic of trauma unless the student believes their character would be trying to bring up the topic to the therapist. Instructors should expect that some issues are more difficult to talk about in a clinical setting, but this is different from dangling clues and waiting for the student-therapist to figure out the reason for some aspect of the character's personality or behavior.

Instructors should ensure that students avoid playing "stump the therapist." Students already working as counselors or therapists may be tempted to role-play an extremely difficult problem, based on their own efforts to understand challenging clinical situations. However, this may set up the therapist/partner with an experience more difficult than intended for the class. The emphasis should be on character accuracy and consistency, rather than an unreasonably challenging task for the student-therapist (Browning & Kabasakalian-Mckay, 1995). Unless it is the point of the exercise, the creation of resistant clients for role-play exercises should be avoided.

## Step 5: Shape the Family Through Continued Discussion

After each participant has created a fully rounded character, the students present their characters to the family. Family members continue to build the family by posing questions to each other, such as: (a) What is our socio-economic status? (b) What is our parents' level of education? (c) Where do we live? (d) What presenting problem brings us to treatment? (e) Who called for treatment? (f) Are we isolated as a family? (g) Do we share a religious belief system? (h) What are family members' jobs, hobbies, pastimes, and outside commitments? (i) How involved are in-laws? The list of questions should not be exhaustive, and should evolve as the family members communicate with each other. The decisions made about the family should not be dominated by one person, and a decision made by one member of the family can be rejected by the others at any time. For example, if one member of the family says, "I'll assume that as the father I have been distant and a little physically abusive over the years," another student may say, "I'm sorry, but I can't tolerate the possibility that my father, in this role-play, is abusive, I'll need that part changed." This component of the process typically takes about two hours.

## Step 6: Create Subsystem "Secrets"

Family subsystems are subsets of family members that have "secrets" unknown to other family members; these include parents, children, a biological parent and his or her biological child, or a parent and an extended family member. Give every subsystem 10 minutes to create subsystem secrets that should not be shared with the whole family. For example, if the "father" character had a drinking problem early in the marriage, this information would be kept secret from the "children" and would be known to only the mother-father subsystem. However, if the "mother" had said during the initial family meeting, "My character had an affair, but let's assume that not everyone knows," this is not a subsystem secret, and the instructor must inform the family that because the affair was revealed to everyone, it must either be dropped or incorporated into general family knowledge. By building the family this way, no character has to pretend not to know something, and students are able to keep secrets within subsystems separate from the others. This exercise is based on honesty in role in order to build responses or reactions that are genuine and realistic.

## Step 7: Create an Intake for the Participating Therapist

One family member should complete an intake form and give it to the therapist. This is simply a paragraph introducing the family to the therapist, and should include standard intake information, such as the names and ages of each family member and the presenting problem.

## Step 8: Spend Time in Role

Before the first session, the family should eat at least one entire meal together "in character," avoiding the temptation to drop the role during the meal. This is of critical importance, because "family" dynamics are developed through interaction during the meal. For example, during the role-play a child character may state to the father character, "Today at lunch I was mad because you were yelling at me about my grades at school." Alternatively, if a husband tells his wife about a situation at work that requires some kind of sacrifice by the family, the mother and/or children may respond in character. In our experience, much material developed during the meal pertains to the presenting problem and is used by the student-therapist during the role-play therapy session.

During role-play, the therapist will invariably pose questions that were not previously considered by the family. On most occasions, spending time in the role supplies enough material for answering such questions and allows the participants to continue the exercise effectively. It also allows members to become more aware of family roles, rules, and styles of interaction, among other things.

## Step 9: Provide Feedback on Family Creation

Continuous feedback throughout the creation process is essential. The instructor should sit with the "family" and listen to them in character before the first therapy session, and pose questions to them to see if they respond as a family might in a clinical setting. If responses seem unrealistic, the instructor should provide clear suggestions to assure role-play authenticity. For example, if the character of a stepfather insists that he loves his stepchildren more than he loves his biological children, the instructor might clarify that such a response, although possible, is so rare that it compromises authenticity.

## Step 10: Undergo the First Family Therapy Session

During the entire first session, the "family" should remain in character and refrain from giving the therapist feedback after the session. The family will provide feedback later in the process during the final debriefing. However, the instructor may offer supervision to the student-therapist at any time in the exercise. Although live supervision technology is preferred during student-therapist meetings with the role-play family, this meeting may be videotaped outside of class and used for subsequent supervision or class presentation. Other students should not discuss the role-play, thus observing the same ethical and confidentiality constraints that would apply to a demonstration session with an actual family.

## Step 11: Prepare for Subsequent Sessions

Before each subsequent session, it is essential for the family to meet out of character outside of class to discuss how each character reacted to the previous session and events. If the therapist assigned any homework to the family, realistic reactions of family members to the assignment should be discussed by students in the family. For example, if the therapist suggested that the family brainstorm about activities they could do together that all members would enjoy, the group should meet and actually brainstorm. Some assignments, like a one-on-one recreational outing with father and child, may be unrealistic for the family to duplicate. However, taking part in these assignments helps students further refine characters, clarify patterns of engagement and communication, and identify emotional responses family members have toward each other.

## Step 12: Supervise Students

As noted, live supervision, via a one-way mirror or closed circuit TV, is strongly recommended in order to make the exercise a more active learning process. After each session, the family is dismissed to work on Step 11, while the instructor offers feedback to the student-therapist. Typically, after asking the student to reflect on the session and providing supportive comments, the instructor reviews the notes compiled during the session and discusses how well the student matches the core clinical competencies (American Association of Marriage and Family Therapists, 2004).

## Step 13: Provide the Final Debriefing to the Family

The final debriefing is of critical importance. Role-playing can generate strong emotions in the student portraying a character. Consequently, during the final debriefing members of the "family" need to discuss honestly and in detail their responses to being in character, the feelings generated by family membership, and their reactions to the different therapists. A student's response to role-play may help identify issues that can be explored through supervision or personal therapy.

## Step 14: Provide Feedback to the Therapist

Although candid feedback to the student-therapist can arouse anxiety and defensiveness, it is an essential part of fostering the development of outstanding clinical skills. To reduce defensiveness and the sense of vulnerability during such a critique, it may be helpful to follow some basic guidelines, such as encouraging students to discuss the strengths and weaknesses of their own work (Erckert, 2002).

After the role-playing is completed, the "family's" feedback to the participating role-play therapist or student-family life educator can be guided by the following questions: What were the positive aspects of the session? Do you have any suggestions about other interventions you might have wanted to make in this session?

With regards to evaluating students, we have generally "graded" their involvement throughout the process as part of the class participation segment of the overall class grade. However, the majority of the course grade is determined by a written self-evaluation in which the students must describe the rationale for specific interventions and offer suggestions for any changes in approach that might be helpful.

## STUDENT REACTIONS

To assess how effectively the protocol increased empathy and developed clinical skills, one of the authors conducted in-depth interviews with eight students to solicit reactions from students who used this protocol during their training. The interviewing process met IRB standards and written notes on student feedback were recorded. The following is a list of questions posed to the students, followed by examples of student responses.

### A. What Did You (the Student) Find Beneficial About Role-Playing a Character?

Regardless of the type of family portrayed, students reported that they gained a level and type of knowledge distinct from that provided by a lecture or reading. One participant commented that, "Role-playing provides a unique opportunity to learn about client difficulties from a personal point of view and experience the range of emotions that take place for a client during a session. Some students also commented on the benefits of having a "safe" environment to try out clinical interventions.

Participants consistently recognized, as the most significant benefit of the protocol, an increase in empathic understanding for the situation faced by the "family." Specific comments from students about increasing empathy are listed under question D, listed below.

## B. What Aspects Were Not Beneficial?

Although most students' reactions were positive, some felt that having different students pose as therapists made the process difficult. One student said, "Beginning each session with a new therapist is difficult and having to repeat demographic intake information many times becomes tiresome. The characters that are developed are quite extensive, and although I made every attempt to be complete and thorough in preparation, I was asked questions that I did not prepare for in advance, which caused some moments of anxiety. It is also easy to respond to similar questions with different responses, simply because you have forgotten what was said in a previous interview."

## C. In What Areas Did You Find the Character Difficult to Portray?

Some students noted difficulties in portraying the real emotions of their characters. A participant remarked, "I am not trained in acting. There were times when I was role-playing that I felt that a certain display of emotion would be appropriate to demonstrate the feelings of grief, anger, or helplessness that my character was experiencing during the session. Upon review of the tape however, I felt that I didn't provide a true representation of emotion that was being experienced."

Another student reported, "I found it difficult to play emotional reactions that were not part of my own personality style. For example, my character needed to react angrily to situations in the family in a way that wasn't natural for me. There were times when I wasn't sure if I was over-reacting or under-reacting emotionally. I can see the need to pick a character that isn't too far removed from your own personality."

## D. Did Portraying This Character Increase Your Empathetic Understanding of a Future Client?

As mentioned above, students overwhelmingly reported an increase in empathic understanding by engaging in this exercise. One student reported, "It is amazing how much understanding I gained from doing this work. The empathetic understanding gained through these role-play experiences leads to, at minimum, a basic understanding of future client problems on a personal level."

Another participant commented, "By interacting with the other family members, I was really able to understand what a client in a similar situation might feel and how she would react than if I hadn't role-played my character. I felt as if I began to really understand her concerns and her situation in the family."

In addition, students reported that the realism of the family led the therapist to honestly care about the "family" in therapy and thus heightened their desire to "do no harm."

### E. What Was Your Reaction to the Feedback Received by Others?

Some participants felt that having an active feedback session with colleagues who were part of the same experience, and who would also be experiencing feedback, led to a feeling of learning from each other and not just competing. One student noted, "Feedback is always anxiety provoking. I know that giving and receiving feedback is a necessary aspect of this profession. Mistakes are going to be made, and strengths are going to be developed. I found that the role-playing experience allowed this all to happen in a safe and supervised environment, which lessened some of my anxiety."

### F. How Has This Experience Contributed to Your Professional Development?

Most students reported that the protocol enabled them to learn and refine new therapeutic techniques. Other participants reported that watching the other students take turns at being the therapist was useful. One participant commented that, "A benefit to portraying a character for several therapists is the ability to experience different styles and interventions for the same problem." Similarly, another student noted that, "When I watched how the various therapists worked with the role-play families, I found that I was more comfortable with some therapeutic styles than others. It was helpful to see that, while my own style might be different from someone else's, I could still be effective."

Students also reported being grateful to have a realistic and workable family in which to practice family therapy techniques. Students also have noted that, because of this experience, they would be more careful not to proceed blithely with topics, and that after role-playing a particular situation (e.g., a stepfamily, a lesbian family or a family with an addiction), they would be more aware of the issues likely to be difficult.

One participant remarked, "As a new therapist, there are many situations and client problems that I had never experienced. The role-playing experience allowed me to apply my learned understanding to new client problems."

## Additional Student Observations and Observations

In addition to the above responses, many of the students reported that their own personal characteristics overlapped with their characters. The characteristics most frequently cited by the students as held in common were: (a) marital status, (b) religious beliefs, (c) educational status, (d) parental marriage status, (e) deceased family member, (f) the presence of children, and (g) selected personality traits. Students often relied on their own life experiences and found it nearly impossible to be different completely from their characters. Although the students generally found the impact to be insignificant, most recognized that it could lead to greater vulnerability if they were conflicted about that aspect of themselves. This indicates that instructors, while acknowledging that drawing from oneself is natural and increases role-play realism, should explicitly reinforce the direction that students assume characteristics or a history that does not completely match their own experiences. Emphasizing this aspect of the protocol both increases the student's empathy for others who are dissimilar and protects the student from revealing personal vulnerabilities. It also may reduce the feeling of being personally attacked during the feedback portion of the protocol.

Finally, the students' perceptions of the value of the Creating Families protocol are consistent with our own observations. We have found the therapy sessions to be extremely lifelike, and the knowledge, empathy, and clinical skills gained by students to be far greater than would be possible from lecture- or tape-based instruction.

## ADDRESSING ETHICAL CONCERNS

Instructors who use this protocol should ensure that students voluntarily consent to engage in this experiential learning process, in adherence to APA Ethical Principles of Psychologists and Code of Conduct (American Psychological Association, 2002). While most students are grateful for the opportunity to benefit from experiential learning that is pertinent to their education, some students may be reluctant to participate in the exercise for a number of reasons. In such cases, instructors might require an alternative written assignment that requires the same time and effort and covers the same topic area as the experiential exercise. Alternatively, the course syllabus could indicate clearly that an experiential learning assignment is a requirement, so by registering for the class, the student is agreeing to participate. This method is particularly useful for elective courses.

While the protocol is designed to protect students by helping them to create a character that does not incorporate too much personal material, the process is one that can, and generally does, produce strong emotions. If the emotions generated are not confined to the "characters" but begin to infiltrate the students themselves, the instructor must be available to discuss any area in which the student requires assistance, or to take students aside if their comments in character appear overly distressing. Of course, the instructor must make appropriate recommendations if the student begins to bring up topics of a clinical nature. The effectiveness of the exercise would be reduced if it resulted in the student feeling overly vulnerable.

Ethical concerns that arise in role-playing typically reflect the tendency of students to view the experience of selecting a character to play as an opportunity to work out a personal problem, or to reflect on an issue presented by a friend or client. Therefore, the "therapy" is altered by needs and perceptions that are not in keeping with the character portrayed. The student-therapist may do the correct intervention, but receive feedback from the role-play family that appears unrealistic to the instructor and other class members. However, it is often difficult for the instructor to challenge a student's interpretation of a character. Moreover, the instructor may suspect that a personal dynamic is overshadowing the depiction of the character, but he or she may not wish to bring that up publicly. The Creating Family protocol decreases the likelihood of the negative aspects of working out a personal response in class because students are given very specific instructions on how and from where to draw the clinical material.

## DISCUSSION

Our experience shows that role-playing a character within a family provides great benefits to the student from both an empathy building and learning perspective. When a student has prepared for the role-play properly, following the protocol described, he or she begins to rely on both the constructed history and the empathy created during the session to maintain the character's beliefs and feelings. Empathy generated during a role-play allows the students to experience strong emotions without necessarily confronting their personal issues. Rather than being directly therapeutic, the student leaves this process with an increased empathetic perspective on a population other than his or her own. In fact, as noted earlier, some students who have participated in the role-play process reported that, after spending time in character, began to experience almost spontaneously a character's defenses, feelings, and responses to a given situation (Collins, 2004). In addition to increasing empathy for the character, the ability to "become" the client allowed for real and lifelike interactions with other members of the family as well as the therapist.

One of the other benefits of the protocol is that as students who are in character begin to experience emotions that surface during the session, they may discover personal traits and skills that are relevant to their growth as a therapist, a family life educator, or a human services professional. For example, a student role-playing a character who was sexually abused as a child may realize that he or she will have difficulty working with such a client professionally because of the role-play experience. Conversely, a student who finds it difficult to empathize with the created character may wish to explore how this difficulty affects professional development or the ability to work with such a client in the future.

Another substantial benefit of the role-playing exercise is that students who assume the role of a family member can gain valuable insight into clinical techniques, when they experience first-hand the emotions and reactions produced by another student therapist. Because the therapy occurs in a constructed context rather than one with real clients, students can learn from successes as well as failures without putting clients at risk. They have the opportunity to understand better which techniques might be effective for a given situation, thus improving their own professional skills.

Tolan and Lendrum (1995) articulated several critical factors that, when addressed successfully, create a useful and authentic role-play. They examined trainee self-awareness and empathy, and developed two procedures to create material that help produce the character's "life." The first was to encourage the students to tap into personal history; the second was to develop "projected" life facts about a non-existent person, which can in turn extend and increase empathy toward people unlike oneself. We believe the protocol described here successfully accomplishes both of these, while protecting students from disclosures that may compromise them or render them vulnerable.

Although this technique has been used exclusively in teaching empathy and clinical skills in the class and in workshops, it certainly may be possible for other teachers to find the technique to be useful in other settings. Certainly Sociologists and Family Life Educators might find such a technique extremely helpful in expanding a student's understanding of alternate family compositions. Once created, the "family" could be placed in front of a class and interviewed as part of a lecture. To date, however, the clinical teaching application has been the primary motivation for this process.

## SUMMARY

Our purpose in developing the "Creating Families" protocol was to enhance the education of student counselors and therapists by utilizing a comprehensive role-play format designed specifically for working with families. We have delineated a protocol that may be used by any instructor who desires to increase the reality of role-play scenarios; and we have reviewed the ethical implications of the process, to help the instructor feel confident that the safety of the student is addressed. A secondary, yet critically important benefit, is the ability of role-plays to enhance the student's empathic understanding of the dilemmas experienced by their "character." By encouraging the development of characters "from the ground up," the described protocol helps facilitate increased realism for both the "family" and the student-therapist. Also, because they gain the experience of having "lived" some of the issues that they are likely to experience in the therapeutic context, students experience and understand an entire range of family concerns. Finally, this protocol provides the instructor with a more realistic therapy session in which to critique the skills of the student-therapist.

## REFERENCES

American Association of Marriage and Family Therapists Core Competencies Taskforce. (2004). *The marriage and family therapy core competencies*. Alexandria, VA: The American Association for Marriage and Family Therapy. Copies available by contacting Bill Northey: bnorthey@aamft.org.

American Psychological Association. (2002). *Ethical principles of psychologists and code of conduct*. Washington, DC: Author.

Banyard, V. & Fernald, P. (2002). Simulated family therapy: A classroom demonstration. *Teaching of Psychology, 29*, 223-226.

Bohart, A. & Greenberg, L. S. (1997). *Empathy reconsidered*. Washington, DC: American Psychological Association Press.

Browning, S. & Kabasakalian-McKay, R. (1995). *Creating families: Training family therapist to work with diversity*. Paper presented at the 24th Annual Mid-Winter Conference of the Eastern Psychological Association, Philadelphia, PA.

Collins, J. S. (2004). Personal communications, August 6.

Erckert, I. M. (2002). *Guidelines for offering feedback of videotaped roleplay.* Presented at graduate level course, Chestnut Hill College, Philadelphia, PA.

Furr, S. & Carroll, J. (2003). Critical incidents in student counselor development. *Journal of Counseling & Development, 81,* 483-489.

Helmeke, K. & Prouty, A. (2001). Do we really understand? An experiential exercise for training family therapists. *Journal of Marital and Family Therapy, 27,* 535-544.

Kim, B. & Lyons, H. (2003). Experiential activities and multicultural counseling competence training. *Journal of Counseling & Development, 81,* 400-408.

Levitov, J., Fall, K., & Jennings, M. (1999). Counselor clinical training with client actors. *Counselor Education & Supervision, 38,* 249-259.

Martin-Smith, A. (1995). Quantum drama: Transforming consciousness through narrative and roleplay. *Journal of Educational Thought, 29,* 34-44.

Rabinowitz, F. (1997). Teaching counseling through a semester-long role play. *Counselor Education & Supervision, 36,* 216-223.

Shepard, D. (2002). Innovative methods: Using screenwriting techniques to create realistic and ethical role plays. *Counselor Education & Supervision, 42,* 145-158.

Tolan, J. & Lendrum, S. (1995). *Case material and role-play in counseling training.* London: Routledge Press.

VanderGraf, L. (1998). Personal communication, March 14.

Yalom, I. (2002). *The gift of therapy.* New York: Harper Collins Press.

# Small-Group Learning and Hypothetical Families in a Large Introductory Course

Tanya Koropeckyj-Cox
Colleen Cain
Justin Coran

**ABSTRACT.** Increased university enrollments and large class sizes, especially at the introductory level, demand creative approaches to promote learning and engagement in the classroom. Small-group work can help achieve these goals, creating a positive and memorable student experience. We propose a small-group exercise that can supplement the traditional lecture format in an introductory marriage and families course. Students are assigned to small groups as members of hypothetical families and are presented with real-life situations over the course of the semester (e.g., job loss or promotion, illness, or extended absence of a family member). Students write about each new situation's effects on their individual character and discuss the implications and potential adjustments for the family. To ensure participation, students who miss

---

Tanya Koropeckyj-Cox is Assistant Professor, Department of Sociology, Colleen Cain is a graduate student, Department of Sociology, and Justin Coran is an undergraduate sociology major, all at the University of Florida.

Address correspondence to: Tanya Koropeckyj-Cox, Department of Sociology, University of Florida, P.O. Box 117330, 3219 Turlington Hall, Gainesville, FL 32611-7230 (E-mail: tkcox@soc.ufl.edu).

The authors thank graduate students Monica Morris, Danielle Dirks, and Gretchen Pendell who assisted with the small-group scenario process and with the Introduction to Marriage and Families course. Also, the authors thank the nearly 1,050 students in the course whose participation has brought the process to life and whose comments and suggestions have contributed to its continual improvement. In addition, the authors are grateful to three anonymous reviewers of this article for their helpful comments.

© 2005 by The Haworth Press, Inc. All rights reserved.
doi:10.1300/J002v38n04_02

class can complete an online version of the assignment. This exercise encourages a critical imagination, promotes interaction and participation, and challenges students to think critically by applying course concepts.

*[Article copies available for a fee from The Haworth Document Delivery Service: 1-800-HAWORTH. E-mail address: <docdelivery@haworthpress.com> Website: <http://www.HaworthPress.com> © 2005 by The Haworth Press, Inc. All rights reserved.]*

**KEYWORDS.** Teaching, group work, scenarios, large classrooms, marriage and family courses

## INTRODUCTION

The demographic effects of large birth cohorts and continued immigration are increasing demand for space in undergraduate courses in many states, especially at public colleges and universities (Hebel, 2004). Total enrollment at American colleges is expected to rise 19 percent between 2000 and 2013, according to recent projections by the U.S. Department of Education (Young, 2003). Even without the population pressures, college and university enrollments are likely to remain high because of the importance of higher education for individual opportunities and for fueling state economies (Hebel, 2004). Increased enrollment means larger courses, especially at the introductory level. Instructors face heightened demands to effectively teach large numbers of students–a tough challenge, though one that can be met with creativity and preparation (Bartlett, 2003).

At the same time, there is a growing interest among educators to move away from traditional lectures typically used in larger courses to more creative formats and methods that engage students through active learning and critical thinking. For example, Sandifer-Stech and Gerhardt (2001) have noted that traditional, lecture-based methods of teaching and learning are being challenged and greater emphasis is being placed on interactive student learning through case studies, debates, personal letters, and simulation exercises.

The current article describes a small-group classroom activity in which students are divided into hypothetical families. The exercise stresses active learning and student interaction within the context of a large (150 student) introductory marriage and families course taught in a large lecture hall (and without smaller discussion sections). We propose a framework that helps to structure individual learning, small-group discussion, and interaction within the larger classroom. Continually updated and refined, this framework allows considerable flexibility in adapting to different instructor preferences, technological tools, student interests, and larger societal issues. We begin with a brief summary of the literature on group work and active learning. We then explain the goals and objectives of the exercise and describe the process, including its preparation and execution. We conclude by discussing the merits and caveats of the process based on seven semesters of its implementation and refinement.

## *LITERATURE REVIEW AND OBJECTIVES*

Research on small group work and active learning in the classroom has overwhelmingly reported positive student response. Active learning approaches, in which students actively examine issues while the instructor provides structure and support, can help to enliven classes and promote a deeper understanding of course material (Hamlin & Janssen, 1987). Active learning approaches include cooperative learning and collaborative learning. Cooperative learning specifically involves both group goals and individual responsibility; students work together in small, interdependent groups to extend or apply material from course reading or instruction (Johnson, Johnson & Smith, 1986; Slavin, 1991). Slavin's (1991) review of research on cooperative learning in elementary through secondary classrooms has found that it enhances academic achievement, intergroup relations, and self-esteem. Others have noted that cooperative learning can help students to learn other viewpoints, mutually support one other, and develop a deeper understanding of their course material (Johnson et al., 1986).

Educators have distinguished between cooperative learning, which is more structured, and collaborative learning, which emphasizes the social context of learning and is less prescriptive or directive to students (Oxford, 1997). A collaborative approach represents a welcome alternative from formal lectures, allowing for discussion, group interaction, and improved student learning (McKinney & Graham-Buxton, 1993). Lehman (1997) suggests that collaborative work encourages students to learn from each other and to participate more actively in class.

Active learning methods have been widely used and evaluated in small classes, but few articles have addressed small group work in the large college classroom setting (i.e., more than 60 students), especially in courses on Marriage and Families. Yet, large classes pose considerable challenges for promoting attendance, participation, and interaction, and the benefits of active learning may be particularly helpful in such settings. McKinney and Graham-Buxton (1993) have found that "group work can reduce anonymity and isolation" (p. 403) and offer a component of the student grade that is "not based on the multiple-choice examinations common in many large classes" (p. 403). Hamlin and Janssen (1987) also have noted that active learning encourages student interaction in class time and fosters greater comprehension of concepts.

Active learning and realistic scenarios can be used in class discussion to promote critical thinking by discussing and applying important concepts through concrete examples. This method helps students to become aware of the link between personal experiences and larger social forces. Through group work, students can hear a variety of perspectives from their peers, allowing them to place their own individual views and experiences in a larger social context. Hypothetical scenarios and other active or collaborative learning exercises have been particularly effective in teaching about diversity and social inequality, including economic and gender stratification (e.g., Hamlin & Janssen, 1987; Lehman, 1997), and McCammon (1999) has specifically integrated considerations of family structure into a scenario exercise on social stratification. Sandifer-Stech and Gerhardt (2001) have used problem-based learning in an undergraduate family studies course, using real-world problems or situations to focus in-class learning; though their procedure was more structured and intensive than the one we describe below, their findings have reinforced the benefits of creative and interactive learning models.

## *Objectives*

The small-group learning process has been developed in the context of an introductory undergraduate class entitled Introduction to Marriage and Families. With an enrollment of about 150 students each term, the course is taught in a large lecture hall by a full-time faculty member, with help from a graduate teaching assistant. The students range from first-year students to seniors and represent a wide range of majors and interests.

A major goal of the course is to examine families as crucial primary relationships and as social institutions. Students are encouraged to look at seemingly familiar social issues in new ways, moving beyond their own experiences to consider the circumstances of others and the influence of larger social forces (Mills, 1959). In addition, the course is designed to introduce students to the diversity of family structures, experiences, and resources and to raise their awareness of how these variations and inequalities influence their ability to cope with new challenges and circumstances.

The specific objectives of the small group, to explore hypothetical family circumstances, function to supplement and reinforce the course material and to provide a bridge between theoretical concepts and concrete applications. Additional benefits include increased attendance, participation, and interaction as well as stimulating student interest and creativity.

## *METHOD*

The small-group scenario process is comprised of two components–the hypothetical family groups and the specific circumstances that challenge the groups and their members. The process combines elements of problem-solving approaches and role-play, but it is neither a case study nor is it about acting out specific roles or conversations. Instead, we use the individual roles and groups as a critical context for considering the potential effects of the scenarios and the responses of individuals and families to the new challenges. We emphasize both the short-term and more lasting implications as they vary among different family members and across different groups. This process encourages students to consider multiple perspectives, responses, and adjustments as they are shaped by individual and group circumstances.

### *Constructing the Family Groups*

The small groups are constructed around different types of families and households. Approximately 28-30 groups have been constructed during each term, consisting of four to six students each. The groups include married parents with children, single parents, three-generation families, grandparents raising grandchildren, and blended families as well as unmarried, cohabiting gay or heterosexual couples, with or without children. We have also tried out smaller household groups to reflect the current demographic realities of smaller households and more independent living (e.g., single young adults, never-married or single adults in middle or old age) (see Appendix A). These smaller "groups" also help to accommodate students who are absent on the group assignment day; other latecomers have been added as relatives of existing groups who live in separate households. Each term, four or five class periods are devoted to the small-group process. These sessions are written into the course syllabus and are part of the course grade. We note that the course also includes separate, unannounced in-class assignments to promote class attendance more generally throughout the term.

To facilitate the in-class logistics and allow students some choice in the process, students are asked (during the second week of the course) to arrange themselves into groups of four to six members. The groups are then given their family or household structures, designed to represent diverse family structures and household compositions. Constructed in advance, the group sheets list the family or household members and their characteristics, including relationship, age, gender, and occupation (examples are included in Appendix A). In some cases, additional background details are provided, such as length of relationship, sexual orientation, and aspects of prior history, including adoption, infertility, prior divorce, or unemployment.

For the remainder of the first session, students discuss their individual roles and groups and may add details regarding their families' histories and circumstances. Students have elaborated on details such as residential location or neighborhood, type of housing, and occupations and employers. Several groups have also specified the racial or ethnic characteristics of their family groups.

## *The Scenarios*

Subsequent small-group sessions consider specific scenarios that may affect the family groups and their members. Over time, we have developed and refined the following three core scenarios that have been used each semester: job loss or promotion, the potential for a new relationship, and issues around illness and caregiving. We have also created new scenarios in response to course discussions and larger events happening during the semester.

The discussion of job changes has coincided with assigned readings on social class and socioeconomic issues. Groups are randomly assigned to either a job loss or promotion, and students are encouraged to examine both positive and negative effects. For example, job loss can be a significant source of stress and financial strain, but it may also provide additional time to spend with family members or engaging in childcare. Similarly, a promotion can bring economic and personal gains, but it may also place greater demands on a family member's time and energy. Students consider the potential effects on each individual family member and on the group as a whole, and they are asked to identify and discuss the existing resources (e.g., human and social capital and availability of extended kin) that may facilitate or hinder the family's responses and adaptations to change.

New relationships are considered in conjunction with course readings and class discussion on love, dating, and intimacy. This scenario also considers both positive and negative possibilities. Some groups consider a potential new relationship for an unmarried teen, young adult, or more mature adult. In other groups, a married or committed partner in the family encounters a potential new love interest. We avoid implying any actual infidelity, but prompt students to consider (a) possible circumstances in which an alternative prospect may be seen as attractive or tempting, (b) considerations involved in choosing a course of action, and, (c) possible effects on other family members.

The third regular scenario deals with individual and family responses to illness and dependency. We provide 3-4 possible issues to consider, which have included clinical depression, terminal illness, and chronic, degenerative illness, varying the options over time. For example, we included Parkinson's disease in response to Michael J. Fox's public disclosure of having been diagnosed with the disease several years ago. More recently, in the context of Christopher Reeve's death, we have added an acute, disabling injury. For this scenario, we have allowed students in each group to choose which circumstance they would examine. Given the gravity of each option and the potential for student discomfort, we believe that providing choices has allowed students some control over how to deal with topics that may hit close to home in their own personal lives.

With the beginning of the Iraq War in spring 2003, we added a scenario that dealt with the effects of military deployment and homeland security on families. We have since incorporated military and other related occupations among the initial group characteristics, reflecting the ongoing challenge that they represent. In fall 2004, landfall of four hurricanes in Florida in five weeks caused significant disruption on campus and in the lives of students, providing another scenario topic for class discussion. Applying the hurricane experience to their hypothetical families, students could consider the effects of the storms on a variety of families, and they could discuss and compare their own experiences in a broader context. In response, students have appreciated the opportunity to examine and discuss important issues that are relevant in their own lives. For example, despite differing opinions about the wars in Afghanistan and Iraq, concerns about the effects of military involvement, mobilization of personnel, and non-military roles (including homeland security and humanitarian aid workers) are on the minds of many students. The impact of these current events on families provides an important, timely update that complements more general course materials.

Our experiences with the scenarios have included some pitfalls. We have found that some controversial issues or those with strong moral overtones have posed difficult challenges in class. Although some controversy and disagreement is inevitable (and may be desirable) in a course on marriage and families, the objectives of individual critical thinking and small-group discussion require the ability to consider and discuss multiple perspectives. This process has worked best with issues in which a variety of possible choices or outcomes are evident to students. On the other hand, topics that provoke student discomfort or particularly strong convictions, such as an unexpected pregnancy or end-of-life medical decisions, may lead to conflict and emotional reactions that undermine the ability to openly consider other viewpoints. The example of a potential new love interest has also required careful class management; strong opinions about infidelity may preempt discussion before the context and possible reasons can be examined. As sensitive issues are discussed throughout the course, however, we have found that candor and an early discussion of behavioral guidelines help to create a comfortable and respectful classroom atmosphere and lay a positive foundation for the scenario process. Therefore, with some care and creativity, the hypothetical family groups and scenarios may provide a useful framework for discussing more controversial topics as well.

## The In-Class Procedure

The small-group scenario process has been used in class sessions lasting 50 minutes, 75 minutes, and 100 minutes. Based on our experience, the procedure requires no less than 35 minutes to complete. A longer time period allows for a class presentation on the scenario topic beforehand or a more extended discussion afterward. Careful timing and organization are critical in managing the process within the allotted time.

After a brief introduction or a mini-lecture on the topic, the specific scenario is presented to the students who are already sitting with their groups. Students are first asked to write a paragraph describing the effects of the situation on their individual character and the family. Individual writing provides time for introspection and personal engagement with the topic, which in turn facilitate the group discussion. Next, students discuss the scenario with one another and compare their individual reactions. Specific questions regarding the effects of the scenario and the family's options for responding to new circumstances are provided on a slide to help focus the discussion (for examples, see Appendix B). Each group designates a spokesperson to summarize the group's discussion in writing and in the full class discussion.

The remaining class time is devoted to a full class discussion, providing a forum for sharing different perspectives and hearing about the variety of family groups and their unique responses to similar scenarios. We have found that providing sufficient time for class discussion is challenging and requires careful management, but it is well worth the effort. Class discussion serves to integrate the individual and small-group reactions into a larger, shared learning experience. Successful discussions have been engaging, thoughtful, and often humorous as students share and comment on each other's varied families and responses. Comparisons across groups help to highlight the impact of different family resources and circumstances on their ability to adapt to change–similar events, such as a hurricane or job promotion, may be experienced very differently across family groups. Class discussion also brings out further suggestions or concerns, as students question or supplement each other's perspectives and choices. Visual notes, using a blackboard, transparencies, or computer projection with a word processor, help to keep track of details and highlight important concepts.

## *Evaluation, Participation, and Grading*

To encourage participation and taking the process seriously, the small-group scenario process represents a component of the course grade–usually between 7.5 and 10 percent of the grade each semester. Our experience as well as student comments have underscored the importance of assigning at least some point value to the work–students feel that their efforts should be recognized with course credit. Also, students appreciate having a variety of course grade components so that grades do not rely entirely on multiple-choice exams. On the other hand, the time demands and pressures of grading multiple written assignments in a large class are beyond the resources and capacity of many instructors. We have therefore opted to assign grades on a pass-fail basis, providing full credit for completing satisfactory work, defined as a thoughtful response that considers the individual and family in their larger social context. As a result of the pass-fail approach, we have found that students report less pressure, knowing that their specific ideas will not be scrutinized and graded. By minimizing the perceived risks, this approach rewards participation while encouraging creativity and openness.

## Online Supplement

The small-group scenario process is designed to utilize and enhance class time by stimulating discussion and participation. From the first semester, however, we have had to face some challenges posed by student absences and the uncertainties of having small groups depend on each other's attendance and participation. We have therefore designed the process in a way that is flexible and does not depend on full attendance and cooperation to work successfully. Though in-class discussion is a critical component of the learning process, we believe that the value of contemplating each scenario and of integrating the process with course material justifies providing a method for making up missed classes. Students who cannot attend class are provided the option of accessing the instructions online on the day of class, completing the work on their own, and submitting a written reaction by e-mail within 3 business days of the class session. They are required to submit a somewhat longer, two-page reaction, also graded on a pass-fail basis. The longer length requirement has helped to discourage students from doing all of the work individually outside of class. Another option has been to count one e-mailed assignment for full credit (in case of an unavoidable absence), with any subsequent e-mailed assignments given a reduced point value. In seven semesters, however, very few students have submitted more than one missed assignment by e-mail, and each semester has had nearly full participation with about 7 to 9 percent of students submitting e-mailed responses to any given scenario. Thus, the process appears to successfully encourage both attendance and active participation by students.

The use of individual work as the basis for assigning grades has also helped to avoid the "free riding" problem, a recurring theme in critical analyses of group work (e.g., Hamlin & Janssen, 1987; McKinney & Graham-Buxton, 1993). Requiring each student to submit a written reaction has ensured that student grades are independent of the attendance and work of fellow group members. At the same time, conducting the discussions in class, circulating among the groups during small-group discussions, and including time for class-wide discussion have helped to ensure active participation and cooperation in class (see McKeachie, 1999, especially chapters 5, 16, and 19). This process can then be used to reinforce the material from course readings and other class lectures and discussions.

Group work in large classrooms can involve a great deal of work for the instructor and teaching assistant (see McKinney & Graham-Buxton, 1993). This is not something we can easily refute, but several points are worth emphasizing. First, most time consuming is the initial investment in preparing the hypothetical families and constructing the scenario assignments. Once created, the groups and the specific scenario assignments can be refined and adjusted for use in subsequent terms. Second, the exercise can be easily worked into any course covering families (e.g., family policy, family resource management, family diversity, social problems). The overall structure allows for a great deal of flexibility and creativity to adapt to different course constraints and topics. We believe that the benefits of the exercise, including the active engagement in class discussions, are well worth the effort.

## *DISCUSSION*

The small-group scenario process, using hypothetical family groups and real-life family events, emerged out of student suggestions, particularly the individual initiative of one of the co-authors. As a student in the course, Justin Coran approached the instructor and suggested that the course include more opportunities to apply concepts to realistic circumstances. He proposed an overall design and developed the initial model with the instructor (Koropeckyj-Cox). Arising out of a student's perspective, the small-group process represents a valuable bridge between the instructor and students in teaching an introduction to marriage and families.

Over time, we have been impressed with the successes of the process, including almost full participation and the active involvement of students in the context of a large and potentially impersonal class. Students have commented that the group process has helped them to become acquainted with their classmates, a benefit that is particularly valuable in a course that includes many first-year and transfer students making the transition to a large university environment. Many students have also noted that they appreciate being able to compare their perspectives and experiences with their peers. Students are given the opportunity to consider and discuss personally relevant issues with the detachment offered by the use of hypothetical families and scenarios. At the same time, they can "walk in someone else's shoes," gaining a greater understanding of the diversity of family experiences and of the micro and macro factors that shape the circumstances, resources, and potential adaptations of real families.

We have been impressed with the creativity that students have brought to the process. Written work and class discussions have revealed the extensive details that some students and groups have added in an effort to bring their families to life. Some students have brought unique elements of their own experiences into their family characters. For example, without any explicit racial or ethnic characteristics in the assigned families, some groups have personalized their groups by adding these identifiers. In another example, involving the scenario on new relationships, a few students have added details about sexual orientation or past relationships that have stimulated more in-depth discussion of how these issues may influence the meanings and implications of new relationships. These student-initiated changes contribute to the learning process by encouraging their classmates to consider the possible implications of racial-ethnic group, immigration status, or sexual orientation on family dynamics and resources. Though such modifications can be easily incorporated into the design, we find that leaving some room for creativity may help to empower students, encourage a greater level of engagement, and incorporate unanticipated, new perspectives.

At the same time, we have also found that important elements of family diversity need to be specifically identified and developed for students as part of the design. We have experimented with more open-ended guidelines for student groups, allowing them to specify such details as age, relationships, and socio-economic indicators, including occupation. The students in these groups found the process more ambiguous and stressful. Many projected either familiar characteristics or fantasies and clichés onto their families, thus undermining the objectives of exploring diversity and less familiar but realistic experiences. Providing detailed group descriptions has helped students to imagine reality-based families and circumstances very different from their own.

Active learning methods have been criticized for potentially resulting in a loss of factual knowledge, such as names, dates and definitions (Hamlin & Janssen, 1987). By using the small-group scenario process to complement class lectures and readings, our intent is to enhance knowledge through critical thinking and practical application. As we refine the process, however, we are exploring options for anchoring the scenario process more strongly in the factual and conceptual foundations of the course material. Students who have completed scenario assignments online have noted that the additional time and individual nature of their work has encouraged them to seek out relevant readings and to consider the scenarios in greater depth than they would have in class. Based on their suggestions, we envision the potential for adding a student research component (e.g., finding a relevant newspaper article or research article, or informally interviewing friends or family members), either in advance or as part of an individual written reaction completed after class. Another option would be to assign supplementary readings or show related videos that provide substantive details and integrate more general information with specific illustrations from the lives of real families.

Finally, the experience of using the online version of the assignment suggests the potential for adapting the process into a fully online exercise, using out of class group discussion through e-mail or instructional software such as WebCT or Blackboard. However, we caution that such a change could fundamentally alter the nature of the process and its benefits. For example, in-class discussions allow for both small-group and full-class interactions as well as in-person coaching on the part of the instructor and teaching assistant. Further, the in-class process creates a focused interpersonal environment that promotes participation and involvement in the exercise itself and in the class more generally. Adapting the process for use outside of class or in the context of a distance learning course would require additional preparation and careful consideration of how to implement and monitor the group work.

Some students have suggested that the scenario process should represent a more significant course component in terms of both the work involved and the weight for the grade. Several students have also commented on the possibility of using the small-group process as the basis for a larger term project, producing a final group paper and presentation. Such a project would involve additional research and require greater group coordination and cooperation. The downsides include greater risks posed by the uncertainties of student group dynamics and the additional work that would be involved in managing the process, consulting with students, and evaluating their final projects. In somewhat smaller classes or with additional assistants, a more extensive group project can be effective and valuable (see, for example, Hamlin & Janssen, 1987).

We raise a few other cautionary issues that may be helpful in applying this small-group process in other settings. Students learn in different ways and respond to different kinds of exercises and courses. The small-group scenario process works well among students who are comfortable with in-class interactions and with conjuring and discussing hypothetical possibilities. We have found that a few students are reluctant to engage in the process, remaining cynical or detached and completing the minimal requirements for the grade. They take the process less seriously, or they question the value of imagining hypothetical situations. Grounding the process more explicitly in research and in actual family experiences may help to decrease their detachment and skepticism. A second, related challenge is to manage the in-class process to minimize the cynical reactions (e.g., by challenging unrealistic responses among classmates) and reinforce the objectives and insights of the process.

We have found that some kinds of family and household circumstances may present greater difficulty for students. For example, individual roles that involve infants or young children are important to consider, but students have found it difficult to write from that perspective. We have instructed students to think about the scenario as it may influence the child, not necessarily as it is perceived by the child, but many students have gotten stuck on trying to see through the eyes or speak through the voices of very young children. Similar challenges are encountered in considering adults with significant disabilities (e.g., an older adult with Alzheimer's disease or other cognitive disability) or situations in which some family members may not be aware or may not comprehend the problem (e.g., if a married partner meets someone attractive but does not tell anyone). Again, in such cases we have encouraged students to think through the possible ramifications, with or without the individual's full knowledge or understanding of the situation.

Finally, our experience has revealed the importance of presenting a relatively balanced set of scenarios for the family groups. When students perceive the scenarios as "a series of unfortunate events," to borrow the phrase from a children's book series, the potential realism of the hypothetical situations is undermined. This concern relates both to the overall resources and circumstances of the original groups as well as the particular scenarios experienced by the family. Students have found it difficult to imagine adaptations and solutions for these families, eventually resulting in gloomy, fatalistic conclusions and extreme dysfunction. In such cases, class discussion has helped to place these situations in context by including empirical data, case studies or ethnographic accounts that verify their realism and discuss their options. In turn, such discussions provide an opportunity to raise students' awareness of the factors that lead families into difficult circumstances and the social resources that could help them. Some students have also suggested that we incorporate more mundane issues, such as paying bills, managing child care, or negotiating the division of household labor. Common sources of family stress and conflict, these examples may provide less dramatic but realistic considerations of family life.

On a practical level, we note that this exercise has run most smoothly with a teaching assistant or student aide to assist with preparation and with the organizational details of assigning students to groups, distributing the group sheets at the beginning of each scenario session, and helping to manage the small-group discussions. Also, we find that the time of day and the length of class may influence the success of the exercise. The extent and vigor of class discussions reflect student energy levels; late afternoon and Friday classes may be challenging if students are tired or anxious to leave. We have found that scheduling scenarios for Friday afternoons promotes attendance but requires extra effort to encourage student engagement and discussion.

This exercise has worked well when utilized about four or five times over the course of a semester. The sessions supplement class lecture and readings and provide a refreshing break from routine, allowing students to interact and connect with each other. Having fewer than four sessions, especially if spread out over several months, may make it harder for students to remember and relate to their family situations. On the other hand, too many sessions, unless specifically grounded in class topics and additional research may detract from the class material and lose student interest.

Finally, we note that our assessments of this process have drawn on three sources. First, the instructor and teaching assistants discussed our observations of the small-group and class discussions through a debriefing process throughout each semester. Second, we have monitored students' written work for evidence of critical thinking as well as signs of difficulty, frustration, or disengagement. Finally, we have used an open-ended, anonymous student evaluation that asks for reactions and suggestions; students may submit their comments near the end of the term or after final grades have been entered. These methods have served to provide ongoing feedback within the course, but we acknowledge that more systematic evaluation would be valuable to assess the effectiveness of the process as a teaching tool and to identify the circumstances and methods that allow for optimal application.

In conclusion, this small-group scenario process has provided an interesting and engaging method for teaching a 150-student introductory course. We offer our description of the process and of its advantages and pitfalls in order to stimulate further discussion and innovation in the teaching of large college and university courses. As a general framework, this process may be adapted and modified to accommodate different class sizes, disciplinary and conceptual emphases, and technological capacities. The resulting benefits, in terms of individual critical thinking, small-group learning, and full-class discussion, represent a significant enhancement in the teaching of large classes and in the empowerment of students.

## REFERENCES

Bartlett, T. (2003, May 9). Big, but not bad. *The Chronicle of Higher Education.* Retrieved March 25, 2005, from http://chronicle.com/prm/weekly/v49/i35/35a01201.htm

Hamlin, J. & Janssen, J. (1987). Active learning in large introductory sociology courses. *Teaching Sociology, 14,* 45-54.

Hebel, S. (2004, July 2). No room in the class. *The Chronicle of Higher Education.* Retrieved November 8, 2004, from http://chronicle.com/prm/weekly/v50/i43/43a01901.htm

Johnson, D. W., Johnson, R. T. & Smith, K. A. (1986). Academic conflict among students: Controversy and learning. In R. Feldman (Ed.), *Social psychological applications to education* (pp. 199-231). Cambridge University Press.

Lehman, P. (1997). Group problem-solving approach to learning about gender stratification and research process in introductory sociology. *Teaching Sociology, 25,* 72-77.

McCammon, L. (1999). Introducing social stratification and inequality: An active learning technique. *Teaching Sociology, 27,* 44-54.

McKeachie, W. J. (1999). *Teaching tips: Strategies, research, and theory for college and university teachers.* Boston: Houghton Mifflin.

McKinney, K. & Graham-Buxton, M. (1993). The use of collaborative learning groups in the large class: Is it possible? *Teaching Sociology, 21,* 403-408.

Mills, C. W. (1959). *The sociological imagination.* New York: Oxford University Press.

Oxford, R. (1997). Cooperative learning, collaborative learning, and interaction: Three communicative strands in the language classroom. *The Modern Language Journal, 81,* 443-456.

Sandifer-Stech, D. M. & Gerhardt, C. E. (2001). Real world roles: Problem-based learning in undergraduate family studies courses. *Journal of Teaching in Marriage and Family, 1,* 1-17.

Slavin, R. (1991). Synthesis of research on cooperative learning. *Educational Leadership, 48,* 71-82.

Young, J. R. (2003, December 12). Notebook: Enrollment at U.S. colleges will grow 19 percent by 2013, government report says. *The Chronicle of Higher Education.* Retrieved November 9, 2004, from http://chronicle.com/prm/weekly/v50/i16/16a03503.htm

## APPENDIX A
## Sample Family Groups

Here are examples of five groups. Students are provided with the basic family structure, including the ages, genders, and relationships of group members. We also include information on employment and occupation as well as past and potential challenges faced by family members.

**Example Group 1**

| Character | Age | Occupation |
|---|---|---|
| Father- | 45 | Doctor |
| Mother- | 44 | Housewife |

+ 3 children: female (8), female (10), and male (16)

***Important Information About Family:*** The mother and father have been married for 20 years. This is their first marriage, and these are their only children.

**Example Group 2**

| Character | Age | Occupation |
|---|---|---|
| Grandfather- | 65 | Retired |
| Grandmother- | 60 | Employed at home |

+ 3 children, ages 7, 10, and 12

***Important Information About Family:*** The children live with their grandparents. The children's parents died in a car crash five years ago. The grandparents have been married for 39 years and had an only child.

**Example Group 3**

| Character | Age | Occupation |
|---|---|---|
| Father- | 39 | Police officer |
| Mother- | 38 | Computer programmer, unemployed |
| Child-F | 19 | Enlisted, U.S. Army, currently serving in Iraq |

+ 2 more children, ages 12 and 14

***Important Information About Family:*** The mother was laid off from a large company 2 years ago. She has worked in short-term positions but has been unable to find a stable, full-time job.

**Example Group 4**

| Character | Age | Occupation |
|---|---|---|
| Mother- | 45 | Waitress and secretary |

+ 4 children, ages 8, 10, 12, and 17

***Important Information About Family:*** The mother and father divorced 7 years ago, and the mother has custody of their children. The father does not pay child support and has not seen his kids for several years. The mother works two jobs, and the 17-year-old works part-time to help make ends meet.

APPENDIX A (continued)

**Example Group 5**

| Character | Age | Occupation |
|---|---|---|
| Father- | 48 | Car salesman |
| Mother- | 47 | Secretary |
| Grandmother- | 79 | Retired |

+ 2 children, ages 12 and 16

**Important Information About Family:** The grandmother is having increasing difficulty with everyday tasks. She has been recently diagnosed with Alzheimer's disease.

## APPENDIX B
### Sample Scenarios

With each in-class exercise, students are reminded of scenarios that affect families in many ways. As in real life, the effects of these scenarios are not erased; each scenario takes place in the context of the family's problems or successes, resources and vulnerabilities.

**Scenario 1**

The groups are randomly assigned to either scenario 1A or 1B:
1A: A member of the family has lost a job.
1B: A member of the family has been promoted or has been offered a new job with a significant step up in responsibility, work hours, and pay.

**Note:** We restrict the job loss or promotion to adult roles only and to the main earners or potential earners in the family.

Questions to relate to each individual character and to the family group:

1. How does this scenario affect your character?
2. How does this scenario affect the family as a whole?
3. How does the promotion or job loss affect the family's economic resources and future prospects? What changes are likely to result (both positive and negative)?
4. Besides economic changes, how will the family and individual members be affected by the change? (For example, time constraints, child care changes, living arrangements)

In-class discussion focuses on the diversity of family situations and the many ways that families are affected by job changes, including availability of health insurance or other benefits, work hours and extent of flexibility, and longer term career considerations.

## Scenario 2

This scenario deals with health crises and their effects on individuals and family members. Each group may choose one of the options below.

A. A member of the family has been having difficulty lately. After consulting with professionals, the person is diagnosed with clinical depression–treatable with medication and/or therapy, but needing support with daily tasks and stresses.

B. A family member has been diagnosed with terminal cancer with a short prognosis–only 6 months to a year of survival is expected. There is no treatment except to reduce the impact of the symptoms and keep the person as comfortable as possible. The sick family member will need support and daily care.

C. A family member has been diagnosed with Parkinson's Disease. This is a chronic, debilitating disease that slowly increases physical disability. The process may be very difficult emotionally for the person and for the family. Presently there is no cure.

D. A child in the family has been hit by a car and seriously injured. A full recovery is likely, but treatment has involved surgery, several weeks in the hospital, and the need to be immobilized for 8 weeks at home, followed by 3-4 months of physical therapy.

Questions to relate to each individual character and to the family group:

1. Describe who in the family is involved and how this situation will affect him or her.
2. What kinds of challenges does this situation raise for your character? For your family?
3. How will you cope over the *short term*–what kinds of changes or adjustments will you make? What factors might make it harder to cope, or might add to the challenges?
4. How will you cope over the *longer term*? How will the family adjust?
5. What kinds of support from friends or extended family might help your family cope with the situation?

# Psychological Abuse in Family Studies: A Psychoeducational and Preventive Approach

James M. O'Neil
Stephen A. Anderson
Preston A. Britner
Irene Q. Brown
Kathleen Holgerson
Ronald P. Rohner

**ABSTRACT.** One of the first documented psychoeducational programs to educate college students about the perils of psychological abuse is described. The intervention was designed to help students examine their personal experiences of psychological abuse and consider how the information could be used in their careers. The process of creating the intervention and publicizing it to the campus community is discussed. The content of the intervention, participants, implementation, and evaluation processes are described. Operational definitions and dramatic skits of psychological abuse are described along with historical context and current research findings. Ways of working through psychological abuse, and services available to recover from it, are presented. Evaluation data, immediately after workshop completion and one week later, indicated

---

James M. O'Neil, Stephen A. Anderson, Preston A. Britner and Irene Q. Brown are affiliated with the School of Family Studies, Kathleen Holgerson is affiliated with the Women's Center, and Ronald P. Rohner is affiliated with the School of Family Studies and The Rohner Center for the Study of Parental Acceptance and Rejection, all at the University of Connecticut.

Address correspondence to: James O'Neil, School of Family Studies, University of Connecticut, U-2058, Storrs, CT 06269-2058.

© 2005 by The Haworth Press, Inc. All rights reserved.
doi:10.1300/J002v38n04_03

that participants positively evaluated this intervention and reported both positive attitudinal and behavioral outcomes. Limitations and implications of this psychoeducational program for the prevention of interpersonal violence are discussed. *[Article copies available for a fee from The Haworth Document Delivery Service: 1-800-HAWORTH. E-mail address: <docdelivery@haworthpress.com> Website: <http://www.HaworthPress.com> © 2005 by The Haworth Press, Inc. All rights reserved.]*

**KEYWORDS.** Psychological abuse, prevention, psychoeducation, teaching, violence

## INTRODUCTION

Interpersonal violence is an epidemic in America and most societies around the world (American Psychological Association, 1996). Preventive programs are urgently needed to combat child maltreatment, physical violence against women, sexual abuse, elder abuse, and psychological abuse. Preventive and educational programs to decrease these various forms of interpersonal violence are in their early stages of development because little knowledge exists on how to create these interventions. The programs that have been developed are rarely based on theory, research, and evaluation (Geffner, 1997); when they are evaluated, it is only for short-term effects (Crowell & Burgess, 1996).

There are numerous reasons why psychological abuse should be a focus of prevention programs. Psychological abuse may be defined as a pattern of destructive interpersonal behavior that ranges from criticizing to more severe actions that threaten, dehumanize, or treat another as an object rather than a person. Emotional/psychological abuse is often a precursor to physical assault in human relationships (O'Neil & Nadeau, 1999; Stets, 1990). There is some evidence of a cumulative effect when both physical and psychological abuse are present in a relationship (e.g., Zelikovsky & Lynn, 2002). Psychological abuse alone may even be the most destructive and pervasive type of interpersonal violence (Tolman, Rosen, & Wood, 1999; Walker, 1984). No studies support the notion that psychological abuse is *less* harmful than other forms of abuse.

Due to difficulties in defining psychological abuse and methodological problems inherent in assessing it, the actual rate of psychological abuse among children and adults is unknown. More data are available on children exposed to psychological abuse than on adults. Official estimates, based upon child abuse cases reported to social service and legal authorities, suggest that it is the least common form of abuse (U.S. Department of Health and Human Services, 1994). This is likely due to the fact that psychological abuse typically co-occurs with other forms of interpersonal violence, such as physical and sexual abuse or child physical neglect, which are all more easily defined and likely to be reported. However, other evidence presents a different picture. For instance, psychological abuse is the most commonly reported form of child maltreatment among families involved in treatment programs (Daro, 1988). Data from the second National Family Violence Survey indicated that 63% of parents reported engaging in psychological maltreatment toward their children (insulting, swearing, sulking, or refusing to talk) at least once in the past year. The average number of occurrences was almost 13 per year, with 21% reporting more than 20 instances (Vissing, Straus, Gelles, & Harrop, 1991). Female adolescents appear to be at greater risk for psychological abuse than are male adolescents or youth in other age categories (U.S. DHHS, 1994).

Despite evidence of the important correlates and sequelae of psychological abuse, this kind of abuse is taken to be less severe, important, and/or clear cut in definition. Cases of psychological abuse are less likely to be reported to child welfare agencies, teachers, education, and school nurses than cases of physical abuse (Crenshaw, Crenshaw, & Lichtenberg, 1995). Psychological abuse is under-recognized by social service systems, routinely leading to delays in appropriate interventions (Glaser, 2002).

The general public still does not fully understand the effects of psychological abuse. Many people have been psychologically abused, but do not have a vocabulary to describe their experience of maltreatment. Consequently, they struggle to recover from their hurt and are vulnerable to being re-victimized. Given the public's lack of knowledge, psychological abuse is a prime area for educators (e.g., family life educators) to develop preventive educational programs. However, little is known about how to educate people about psychological abuse and how to develop preventive programs that are effective. One critical question that needs to be answered is: Can psychoeducational (or family life education) programs actually help people assess psychological abuse in their lives and deepen their understanding of it personally and professionally?

This paper describes one of the first documented psychoeducational interventions to teach college students about psychological abuse. The college years are an important time to intervene because many young adults are negotiating a multitude of developmental tasks. Chief among these are forming a secure personal and professional identity, managing dating relationships, and establishing intimate and committed relationships that will serve as precursors to future parenting and family relationships.

The intervention was designed to address both the personal experience of psychological abuse and how the topic might be relevant to the career development of students in the helping professions. First, psychoeducation is discussed as the process of using psychological and educational principles and knowledge to help people grow and develop. Second, the process of creating the intervention and systematically publicizing it to the campus community is described. Next, the manuscript describes in detail the content of the intervention, who attended it, and how the program was implemented. The content and process will be described in such a way that readers could replicate the intervention or create their own program in the setting of their choice. Evaluation data on the intervention, immediately after its completion and one week later is presented in the final sections of the manuscript. Finally, the implications and limitations of this psychoeducational intervention for the prevention of interpersonal violence are discussed.

## PSYCHOEDUCATION:
## A CONTEXT FOR PREVENTING PSYCHOLOGICAL ABUSE

Psychoeducation has a 30-year history (Alschuler & Ivey, 1973; Bloom, 1996; Mosher & Sprinthall, 1973) in a variety of educational and mental health settings (see Ripley & Worthington, 2002). In developing our intervention, we defined psychoeducation as a pedagogical approach that uses psychological and learning principles to promote personal, emotional, and intellectual development. Psychoeducation focuses on both the cognitive and affective domains of learning (Bloom, 1956; Krathwohl, Bloom, & Masia, 1964), implying that feelings and emotions have equal weight with conceptual and factual knowledge. For example, Goldberg-Arnold, Fristad, and Gavazzi (1999) discuss a multi-family psychoeducation group that provides families with information, coping skills, and access to social support as mechanisms for improving family and child functioning. With psychoeducation, participants are introduced to multiple contexts in order to fully understand the topic.

Furthermore, positive expectancies are established and multiple learning stimuli are presented to activate participants' thinking and feeling. Participants are invited to be active rather than passive learners. They are engaged experientially and asked to personalize both the content and process of the learning. Psychoeducation also involves helping participants work through any painful memories or events that are activated by the intervention.

Psychoeducation and family life education are interrelated, share common goals and processes, and value program evaluation that assesses learning outcomes (Adler-Baeder & Higginbotham, 2004; Hughes, 1994). Family life education provides individuals and families with educational programs that address a host of prevention and intervention topics (Arcus, 1992; Hughes, 1994).

The preventive intervention described in this paper was based on many of the above principles of psychoeducation and family life education. Specifically, the creators of the program used available data on the prevalence of psychological abuse to anticipate that many students had been victims of this kind of abuse and could still be experiencing negative effects in their lives. Both the cognitive and affective domains of learning were targeted goals of the intervention. This was accomplished by encouraging students to personalize the information on an emotional level using an emotional vocabulary and to think about the academic concepts presented during the program. Positive expectancies were set so that the program could raise consciousness about abuse, foster personal growth, and help people heal from any wounds that they had experienced. Multiple contexts were introduced by presenting information from live skits, psychological theories, empirical research, and historical knowledge. These personal and professional contexts were consistently mentioned to help students see how they could use the information. Stimulus diversity involves alternating the learning stimuli and instruction to touch as many senses as possible (O'Neil, 2001). In this case, the multiple approaches of lectures, live performances, self-assessments, music, and question and answer exchanges facilitated the learning processes.

## *METHOD*

### *Program Preparation Process*

The psychoeducational intervention was entitled "Working With Emotional/Psychological Abuse" and was part of the School of Family Studies, University of Connecticut, Spring 2002 Prevention Series. The Family Violence Initiative (FVI) sponsored the intervention. The FVI is a working group of faculty, graduate students, and Women's Center staff who meet monthly to discuss family violence theory and research. The group also offers service programs educating the university community to the societal and personal aspects of violence. The FVI represents six different disciplines including developmental and counseling psychology, anthropology, women's studies, history, and marriage and family therapy. Therefore, the work of the FVI in creating the psychoeducational intervention was highly interdisciplinary.

Over a period of six months, the FVI group discussed the goals, purposes, funding, publicity, and the proposed outcomes of the intervention on psychological/emotional abuse. The design of the program, methods of implementation, and evaluation processes were arrived at by using consensus decision-making. Careful attention was given to the workshop design because it was assumed that the intervention could be emotionally charged for some of the participants. The group decided that there was a need to have a psychologist available during the program in case any individual needed immediate and special attention.

Faculty colleagues were solicited to help promote the symposium in their classes. Nine faculty members included some aspect of prevention or psychological abuse in their class by giving lectures on the topic, requiring writing assignments related to the topics, or giving class credit for attending the program. These activities gave the concept of psychological abuse more extensive exposure and heightened awareness of the personal and professional issues involved.

## *Publicity and Participants*

The program was advertised through the campus media, and approximately 220 students attended the program in a large auditorium. Although the program was open to the larger campus community, most of the participants (91%) were women. All participants were given a packet of information that included a handout for each part of the program, a psychological abuse self-assessment checklist, and also a program evaluation form.

## *Description of the Psychoeducational Intervention*

The content and process of the two-hour intervention were conceptualized into eight separate, but inter-related parts including: (1) introduction of the program; (2) definition of psychological abuse; (3) audience assessment of psychological abuse; (4) working through psychological abuse: the wounded person cycle and approaches to healing; (5) research on psychological abuse; (6) historical perspectives on psychological abuse; (7) services available to help with psychological abuse; and (8) question and answer period. Each of these is described below.

*Introduction of the program.* The leaders welcomed the participants by communicating the potential value of the program. They discussed the importance of the topic and how "close to home" the issue of emotional/psychological violence is to everyone attending. The audience was encouraged to personalize the program in their lives.

*Definition of psychological abuse.* The definition of psychological abuse presented to the symposium participants was derived from a review of available references in the literature (American Professional Society on the Abuse of Children, 1995; Barnett, Miller-Perrin, & Perrin, 1997; Crossen-Tower, 2002; Tolman et al., 1999) and a vigorous exchange of different ideas among the members of the FVI. Psychological abuse was defined as a pattern of destructive interpersonal behavior that impairs an individual's sense of well-being. This may include mild forms of day-to-day criticism, repeated contradiction, or belittling that leaves the person feeling minimized, devalued, unappreciated, or unjustly treated. Or, it may involve more severe actions that dehumanize or treat another as an object rather than a person. The intent is often to maintain control, advantage, or position over the other. The result is to destroy or impair a person's sense of competence, self-esteem, happiness, and dignity as a human being. It occurs at all stages of the life span and may include any of the following:

- Terrorizing: Verbally assaulting or threatening the individual; creating a climate of fear; bullying; frightening; making the individual believe that their world is hostile and dangerous.
- Spurning (ignoring): Refusing to acknowledge the individual's significance; being unresponsive to the person's emotional (or physical) needs; giving the person the silent treatment; ignoring the person; failing to keep promises or commitments; not appreciating the person's accomplishments, interests, or contributions.
- Devaluing: Making someone feel less competent, inadequate, or less human; humiliating or degrading the person; using verbal put-downs, insults, name-calling, or criticisms of a person's abilities.
- Isolating: Cutting the individual off from normal social experiences; preventing the person from forming friendships; making the person believe that he or she is alone in the world.

Although the focus of the symposium was on experiences of victimization, participants were also encouraged to consider the likelihood that all of us, at one time or another, may engage in psychologically abusive behaviors towards others. It was explained that psychological abuse is not always overt, but can be quite subtle. This definition of psychological abuse provided a context for the entire program. Participants listened to the definition of abuse, observed it on an overhead, and had a copy of it in their packet of handouts. Furthermore, the definitions came to life through the use of dramatic skits.

Students personalized the issues of psychological abuse by observing skits that illustrated the four dimensions of psychological abuse. Four graduate students and one faculty presenter created skits that depicted the conceptual dimensions of terrorizing, spurning, devaluing, and isolating, described above. The relationships portrayed in the skits included a father and pre-teen daughter, a mother and eight-year-old daughter, two female student peers, and male and female partners in a dating relationship. The skits provided participants with specific examples of psychological abuse and were intended to deepen their understanding of how psychological abuse operates in a variety of interpersonal relationships. The skits also were designed to prepare them for their own self-assessment as described below.

*Audience assessment of psychological abuse.* With the above skits and definitions in mind, the audience was asked to make a personal assessment of psychological abuse from their past or present by completing an Emotional/Psychological Abuse Assessment Checklist designed specifically for this workshop. The audience was told that this checklist was an attempt to help each participant personalize the issue of psychological abuse. The checklist included 11 statements about psychological abuse that were derived from the conceptual definition of abuse described earlier. The directions to the checklist were the following: "Below are dimensions of psychological abuse. Using the scale below, rate the degree that you have experienced psychological abuse in the *past* or *present*." A four-point Likert-type scale, ranging from Very Often (4) to Never (1), was used.

This assessment lasted about seven minutes while classical music filled the auditorium. This brief, self-reflection period was used to transition to the next part of the symposium on overcoming psychological abuse.

*Working through psychological abuse.* This part of the intervention focused on how to work through psychological pain using The Wounded Person Cycle conceptualization (O'Neil, Davison, Mutchler, &

Van Buren, 2005). The presenter indicated that there are no prescriptions, quick fixes, or set formulas on how to work through psychological abuse because each person's situation is different. The wounded person cycle involves seven sequential processes for an individual experiencing the wounds of psychological pain. These processes include: (1) injury, violation, and victimization; (2) initial shock, anger, rage, grief, loss, confusion, and emotional pain; (3) initial quest for understanding why the injury happened; (4) development of distorted schemas and activation of defense mechanisms; (5) development of grudges and the telling of one's grievance story; ongoing attributions to explain the injury; blaming the other person and blaming self; (6) rehearsal of the hurt, injury and negative thoughts about the offender; and (7) becoming bonded in the negative, including reoccurring negative emotional outcomes including anger, rage, hate, fear, depression, anxiety, shame, and guilt.

This cycle was explained as repeating itself in the wounded person regularly or when the person feels vulnerable during situational events in their lives. The working through process was described as occurring under three conditions. First, there is recognition that the injury has permanently and negatively changed the person and therefore has left an indelible mark. Second, there is recognition that the old strategies used to escape the wounded person cycle are not producing resolution or closure. Finally, the person considers some other approaches to healing their wounds and working through the hurt. A host of strategies for working through psychological abuse and promoting healing were also presented (O'Neil et al., 2005).

*Research on psychological abuse.* A faculty member provided a brief verbal summary of research regarding the common effects of psychological abuse. Recent research reveals that psychological abuse is as damaging as other forms of abuse (e.g., Hart, Binggeli, & Brassard, 1998). Extensive cross-cultural research finds that, universally, humans respond similarly to psychological abuse in the form of perceived rejection (for an extensive review, see Rohner & Britner, 2002). Psychological abuse tends to lead to psychological maladjustment, including problems with anger, anger management, hostility, and aggression, emotional instability and unresponsiveness, low self-esteem, depression or depressed affect, anxiety and insecurity, substance abuse, conduct problems and behavior disorders among other outcomes (Rohner & Britner, 2002). Participants also were given several handouts that summarized this evidence and suggested research-related readings on the topic.

*Historical perspectives on psychological abuse.* One of the faculty presenters (an historian) gave perspectives on psychological abuse from an historical perspective. The presenter indicated that there has been limited historical analysis of how psychological abuse has evolved and existed over the centuries. Public court records from the nineteenth century documented family members' abusive domination of others. Historical sources from this era also provide evidence of domestic tyranny and communal efforts to control or restrict abusers' oppressive impulses (Brown & Brown, 2003; Pleck, 1987) and the politics of family violence between 1880 and 1960.

*Services available to help with psychological abuse.* A faculty member introduced the idea that there is a solid research base in support of the use of crisis services to meet basic needs immediately, cope in the short-term, and even for long-term changes in the quality of life. As one example, he cited an experimental evaluation by Bybee and Sullivan (2002) that supported the efficacy of a community-based advocacy program for women with abusive partners. The intervention first resulted in connecting the women with community resources and building a network of social support. The women were empowered, and they felt better about themselves. At a two-year follow-up, they were less likely than a comparison group to have experienced any further abuse. In the short run, the important thing was the use of the crisis and advocacy intervention services. In the long run, what was important was that the women felt empowered and saw a change in quality of life-above and beyond the direct effects of services.

The Director of the Women's Center then reviewed the university's Community Response Team information sheet, which lists campus resources (counseling, residence life, Dean of Students, mental health services, health services, the Women's Center and Violence Against Women Program, and the police) and local resources (sexual assault crisis services, domestic violence services). Another handout, "Additional Resources in Connecticut for Working with Psychological Abuse," provided phone and Internet details for the state's database on health and human services, coalition against domestic violence, and coalition of sexual assault crisis services. She noted that most of the services are applicable for intervening with and coping with psychological abuse, in addition to other forms of abuse (e.g., physical or sexual), which may or may not accompany the emotional abuse. The final 30 minutes of the intervention was devoted to questions, answers, and dialogue among the presenters.

## RESULTS

### Evaluation at Program Completion

Surveys were distributed immediately after the intervention to those audience members who remained through the question and answer period. Participants completed the anonymous 11-item questionnaire asking them to evaluate the effectiveness of the program. The exit questionnaire used a four-point Likert scale of 1 (Strongly Disagree), 2 (Disagree), 3 (Agree), and 4 (Strongly Agree). Percentage agreement was calculated by adding the Agree and Strongly Agree responses for each question. The exit evaluation was completed by 127 of the 220 audience members who were present for any part of the symposium. The respondents included 115 females and 12 males. Ninety-four percent were undergraduate students, primarily Human Development and Family Studies and other social science majors.

The results of the evaluation immediately after the intervention are found in Table 1. Ninety percent or more of the respondents agreed that the presenters' ideas were communicated effectively, they learned something valuable, received important information on where to get help with psychological abuse, and that the skits were an effective way to illustrate psychological abuse. Almost as many agreed that the symposium raised their consciousness about abuse in their own lives (85%) and helped them personalize how they had been hurt by psychological abuse in the past or present (71%). These data also indicated that the program stimulated them to learn more about the topic (69%). Finally, a majority of respondents indicated that the program helped them think about enrolling in courses on psychological abuse (64%), and some agreed that the symposium had opened up some possible career options for them (24%).

Furthermore, participants were asked to answer True or False to the following statement: "Emotional/psychological violence can be as harmful as physical or sexual violence." They were also asked "Why? (Please explain your response)." Ninety-four percent of respondents answered "True," while 3% answered "False." The 3% answering false explained that psychological violence often had a longer and/or more harmful impact than other forms of abuse. Three percent did not respond to the question. Thus, *no* participants responding to the evaluation considered psychological violence to be less harmful than physical or sexual abuse. This provided one specific measure of the impact of the symposium. In this anonymous forum, audience members were con-

TABLE 1. Participant Agreement on Ten Evaluation Items Immediately After the Intervention

| % Agreement | Item |
|---|---|
| 94 | The symposium presenters communicated their ideas effectively. |
| 93 | The symposium helped me see where I can get some extra help on campus with psychological/emotional abuse. |
| 90 | I learned something valuable in this symposium on psychological/emotional abuse. |
| 90 | The skits by the graduate students were an effective way to help define what psychological/emotional abuse is really about. |
| 85 | The symposium raised my consciousness about the importance of abuse in my life. |
| 73 | The self-assessment checklist on psychological/emotional abuse helped me personalize how I have been hurt in the past and/or present. |
| 71 | The symposium sensitized me to how I have been hurt by psychological/emotional abuse. |
| 69 | This symposium on psychological/emotional abuse has stimulated me to learn more on this topic. |
| 64 | This symposium has made me want to enroll in further course work, workshops, or programs related to psychological/emotional abuse. |
| 24 | This symposium on psychological/emotional abuse has opened up some possible new career roles for me. |

vinced by the symposium–or had pre-existing beliefs confirmed–of the impact of psychological abuse. This finding is impressive given the lack of recognition of psychological abuse in the general population and chronic under-reporting by educators and medical and child welfare professionals (Crenshaw et al., 1995; Glaser, 2002).

Positive qualitative comments written on the questionnaires included: "informative," "enjoyable," "enlightening," and "wonderful!"; "handouts were useful"; "well organized"; "dialogue at end was very helpful"; "sparked my interest and led me to look at my own life"; and, "I appreciated that you included the resource component and had someone available for talking to (resources; available counselor)." On the negative side, several participants disliked the self-assessment questionnaire and the skits, but they did not indicate why.

## Evaluation One Week Later

An 8-item questionnaire was administered to 127 (58%) of those attending one week after the intervention. The second evaluation focused on attitudinal and behavioral outcomes of the intervention. Using the following stem for each item, "Because of the symposium last week," respondents reported their thoughts and behaviors related to psychological abuse. The results indicated that the participants were affected by the intervention one week later. See Table 2. In percentages ranging from 60-87 percent, the respondents agreed that (1) their consciousness had been raised, (2) they had thought more about psychological abuse and the ideas presented in the workshop, (3) they had considered how psychological abuse occurred in their own lives, and (4) they had heard or observed something that made them think about the symposium.

Qualitative, open-ended comments at follow-up mirrored the positive adjectives from the earlier assessment. Students wrote that the symposium: "helped me realize abuse in my own life and made me think about how I can maybe change it"; "made me recognize my roommate's situation with her boyfriend as emotional abuse"; "made the topic of emotional and psychological abuse much more real to me." One participant commented that, "I see a lot of psychological abuse in relationships (romantic) and I took some of the handouts we got about it and made copies to give to people in hopes of raising awareness."

## DISCUSSION

The results indicated that the intervention was successful in educating college students about the topic of psychological abuse. Participants who completed the evaluation survey indicated that the program raised their consciousness about the prevalence of psychological abuse, helped them to recognize the actual dynamics of psychological abuse, and was useful in directing them to sources of help for coping with abuse. The self-assessment checklist appeared to be a useful tool in helping participants to personalize the psychological abuse concept, even in a large auditorium setting. Respondents also reported that the intervention stimulated them to learn more about psychological abuse in future courses, and about one quarter of them indicated that some new career roles had been opened up by the presentations. The follow-up assessment one week later indicated that thinking about psychological abuse continued after the intervention for more than half of those

TABLE 2. Participant Agreement on Eight Evaluation Items One Week After the Intervention

| % Agreement | Items ("Because of the symposium, over the last week:") |
| --- | --- |
| 87 | I feel that the symposium raised my consciousness about the importance of psychological/emotional abuse. |
| 74 | I have thought about an idea that was presented during the symposium. |
| 68 | I heard or observed something that made me think about the symposium. |
| 68 | I have thought more about the topic of psychological/emotional abuse. |
| 63 | I have discussed psychological/emotional abuse with at least one other person. |
| 62 | I have thought more about psychological/emotional abuse in my personal life. |
| 56 | I have thought about a possible career that relates to psychological/emotional abuse. |
| 55 | I have initiated a conversation about psychological/emotional abuse with another person. |

polled. Fifty percent of the respondents reported having conversations with others about psychological abuse during the week following the program.

There are limitations to the intervention and how it was evaluated. Foremost, the evaluation design could have been more systematic and sophisticated. A control group and randomization of subjects would have allowed for an experimental testing of the intervention. This more rigorous experimental study is recommended for future research when teaching about psychological abuse. Furthermore, a follow-up period of longer than one week could have documented whether the program had any long-term effects. The use of a simple, self-report evaluation questionnaire failed to assess the personal and emotional reactions to the program. The follow-up questionnaire could have been more precise about how the intervention affected the participants behaviorally and emotionally over time. Additionally, there was no attempt to understand collectively the participants' self-assessments of psychological abuse by openly discussing their responses to the Psychological/Emotional Abuse Assessment Checklist. Given the size of the group, we decided not to have extensive reflection period or discussion of their checklists during the program. We also did not collect these checklists and were therefore unable to determine how many participants viewed themselves as victims of psychological abuse, when such perceived abuse had occurred, who committed the offenses, and the chronicity of the abuse. Finally, because the audience consisted primarily of female, undergraduate students, studying in the social sciences, it is difficult to generalize about the effectiveness of the workshop beyond this population.

The strengths of the program were that it was strategically planned, theoretically based, and included a post-workshop evaluation and follow-up. Faculty and staff from six different professions created the psychoeducational intervention and consequently the program had interdisciplinary depth and comprehensiveness. The psychoeducational model provided a theoretical foundation for planning and implementing consciousness-raising around a sensitive topic like psychological abuse. Furthermore, providing participants with services to resolve their abuse and having a psychologist available in the audience for immediate attention, gave the program a dimension of concern and care. The extensive printed handouts dispersed to participants gave them an opportunity to study psychological abuse after the program ended. Connecting the intervention to different academic classes in the School of Family Studies and using the campus media proactively promoted the concept of psychological abuse to the larger campus community.

Using stimulus diversity techniques of self-disclosure, live performances, movie clips and music videos, and self-assessment checklists can help participants personalize and process psychological abuse in diverse ways. We recommend experimentation with different group sizes, with both mixed and same sex groupings, and with different lengths of the program time. For example, our intervention did not allow for extensive personal processing of the participants' self-assessment or the career implications of psychological abuse because of the group size and the design of the program. Our program may have been improved with more time devoted to helping participants discuss their self-assessments and career questions in a large or small group setting. This extended processing time could have increased the program's personal effects and value. Likewise, we recommend greater attention be given to the next steps for participants after psychoeducational programs are concluded. We did provide information on ways to heal and how to access therapeutic services on campus and in the larger community. The program may have been even more useful if specific information was provided on how to cope with the immediate emotional responses of the self-assessment exercise, particularly if participants discovered they had been victimized during the program. For example, the typical emotional responses to just discovering one's own psychological abuse could have been explained. Suggestions could have been made on how to deal with the immediate feelings and thoughts in terms of mobilizing one's coping resources, particularly if one feels alone, vulnerable or angry.

One other consideration not discussed in our program was the importance of individual differences, diversity factors, and how societal oppression affects people's perceptions about psychological abuse and emotional healing. Future programs should provide contexts to understand how sex, race, class, age, ethnicity, sexual orientation, and any other diversity factor, may affect working with psychological abuse. Very little is known about how these diversity factors impact people's experience of psychological abuse.

Knowledge about psychological abuse is in the earlier stages of development, but there is little doubt that this form of maltreatment is widespread and causes pain, suffering, and human wounds that result in significant mental health problems including depression, anxiety, and low self-esteem, to name a few. There is enough known about psychological abuse to educate the public through preventive and psychoeducational programs. We encourage family life educators and other professionals to devote their knowledge and energy to moving this timely and important work forward.

## REFERENCES

Adler-Baeder, F. & Higginbotham, B. (2004). Implications of remarriage and stepfamily formation for marriage education. *Family Relations, 53*, 448-458.

Alschuler A. S. & Ivey, A. E. (1973). Getting into psychological education. *Personnel and Guidance Journal, 51*, 682-691.

American Professional Society on the Abuse of Children. (1995). *Psychosocial evaluation of suspected psychological maltreatment in children and adolescents. Practice guidelines*. Oklahoma City, OK: APSAC.

American Psychological Association. (1996). *Violence and the family report of the American Psychological Association Task Force on Violence and the Family*. Washington, DC: American Psychological Association.

Arcus, M. E. (1992). Family life education: Toward the 21st century. *Family Relations, 41*, 390-393.

Barnett, O. W., Miller-Perrin, C., & Perrin, R. D. (1997). *Family violence across the lifespan*. Thousand Oaks, CA: Sage.

Bloom, B. S. (1956). *Taxonomy of educational objectives: The classification of educational goals. Handbook I: Cognitive domain.* New York: David McKay Company, Inc.

Bloom, M. (1996). *Primary prevention practices.* Thousand Oaks, CA: Sage Publications.

Brown, I. Q. & Brown, R. D. (2003). *The hanging of Ephraim Wheeler: A story of rape, incest, and justice in early America.* Cambridge, MA: Harvard University Press.

Bybee, D. I. & Sullivan, C. M. (2002). The process through which an advocacy intervention resulted in positive change for battered women over time. *American Journal of Community Psychology, 30,* 103-132.

Crenshaw, W. B., Crenshaw, L. M., & Lichtenberg, J. W. (1995). When educators confront child abuse: An analysis of the decision to report. *Child Abuse & Neglect, 19,* 1095-1113.

Crossen-Tower, C. (2002). *Understanding child abuse and neglect (5th ed.).* Boston: Allyn & Bacon.

Crowell, N. A. & Burgess, A. W. (1996). *Understanding violence against women.* Washington, DC: National Academy Press.

Daro, D. (1988). *Confronting child abuse: Research for effective program design.* New York: Free Press.

Geffner, R. (1997). Looking toward the future. In O. W. Barnett, C. Miller-Perrin, & R. D. Perrin (Eds.), *Family violence across the lifespan* (pp. 273-296). Thousand Oaks, CA.: Sage Publications.

Glaser, D. (2002). Emotional abuse and neglect (psychological maltreatment): A conceptual framework. *Child Abuse and Neglect, 26,* 696-714.

Goldberg-Arnold, J. S., Fristad, M. A., & Gavazzi, S. M. (1999). Family psychoeducation: Giving caregivers what they want and need. *Family Relations, 48,* 411-417.

Hart, S. N., Binggeli, N. J., & Brassard, M. R. (1998). Evidence for the effects of psychological maltreatment. *Journal of Emotional Abuse, 1,* 27-58.

Hughes, R. J. (1994). A framework for developing family life education programs. *Family Relations, 43,* 74-80.

Krathwohl, D. R., Bloom, B. S., & Masia, B. B. (1964). *Taxonomy of educational objectives: The classification of educational goals. Handbook II: Affective domain.* New York: David McKay Company, Inc.

Mosher, E. & Sprinthall, N. (1973). Psychological education in secondary schools: A program to promote individual and human development. *American Psychologist, 25,* 911-924.

O'Neil, J. M. (2001). Promoting men's growth and development: Teaching the new psychology of men using psychoeducational philosophy and interventions. In G. E. Good & G. R. Brooks (Eds.), *The new handbook of psychotherapy and counseling with men: A comprehensive guide to settings, problems, and treatment approaches, Vol. 1 & 2* (pp. 639-663). San Francisco, CA: Jossey-Bass.

O'Neil, J. M., Davison, D., Mutchler, M., & Van Buren, J. (2005). *Process evaluation of teaching forgiveness in a workshop and classroom setting.* Manuscript submitted for publication, University of Connecticut.

O'Neil, J. M. & Nadeau, R. (1999). Men's gender role conflict, defense mechanisms, and self-protective defensive strategies: Explaining men's violence against women from a gender-role socialization perspective. In M. Harway & J. M. O'Neil (Eds.), *What causes men's violence against women?* (pp. 89-116). Thousand Oaks, CA: Sage Publications.

Pleck, E. (1987). *Domestic tyranny: The making of American social policy against family violence from colonial times to the present.* New York: Oxford University Press.

Ripley, J. S. & Worthington, E. L., Jr. (2002). Hope-focused and forgiveness-based group interventions to promote marital enrichment. *Journal of Counseling and Development, 80,* 452-463.

Rohner, R. P. & Britner, P. A. (2002). Worldwide mental health correlates of parental acceptance-rejection: Review of cross-cultural and intracultural evidence. *Cross-Cultural Research: The Journal of Comparative Social Science, 36,* 16-47.

Stets, J. E. (1990). Verbal and physical aggression in marriage. *Journal of Marriage and the Family, 52,* 501-514.

Tolman, R. M., Rosen, D., & Wood, G. C. (1999). Psychological maltreatment of women. In R. T. Ammerman & M. Hersen (Eds.), *Assessment of family violence (2nd ed.)* (pp. 322-340). New York: John Wiley.

U.S. Department of Health and Human Services. (1994). *Child maltreatment 1992: Reports from the states to the National Center on Child Abuse and Neglect.* Washington, DC: U.S. Government Printing Office.

Vissing, Y. M., Straus, M. A., Gelles, R. J., & Harrop, J. W. (1991). Verbal aggression by parents and psychosocial problems of children. *Child Abuse and Neglect, 15,* 223-238.

Walker, L. E. (1984). *The battered woman syndrome.* New York: Springer.

Zelikovsky, N. & Lynn, S. J. (2002). Childhood psychological and physical abuse: Psychopathology, dissociation, and Axis I diagnosis. *Journal of Trauma & Dissociation, 3,* 27-58.

# Process Evaluation of Teaching Forgiveness in a Workshop and Classroom Setting

James M. O'Neil
Diane Davison
Matthew S. Mutchler
Jennifer Trachtenberg

**ABSTRACT.** Forgiveness is a process that assists people in releasing their anger, resentment, and negative emotions towards those who have hurt them. This study reports a process evaluation of a psychoeducational workshop and classroom adaptation designed to teach students about forgiveness. We describe the workshop's content, process, and resources in detail. Participants were assessed before, during, and after the workshop across five process areas. The results indicate that the forgiveness workshop and classroom intervention were effective in teaching forgiveness skills, were emotionally challenging, and difficult for some participants because of their pain, confusion, and unanswered questions. We conclude with specific recommendations for improving forgiveness workshops and classroom interventions. *[Article copies available for a fee from The Haworth Document Delivery Service: 1-800-HAWORTH. E-mail address: <docdelivery@haworthpress.com> Website: <http://www.HaworthPress.com> © 2005 by The Haworth Press, Inc. All rights reserved.]*

**KEYWORDS.** Forgiveness, teaching, interventions, evaluation, college students

---

James M. O'Neil, Diane Davison, Matthew S. Mutchler, and Jennifer Trachtenberg are all affiliated with the University of Connecticut.
Address correspondence to: James M. O'Neil, School of Family Studies, University of Connecticut, U-2058, Storrs, CT 06269-2058 (E-mail: James.O'Neil@uconn.edu).

## INTRODUCTION

Forgiveness is a universal, human concept that has existed throughout centuries in nearly all world religions (Rye, Pargament, Ali, Beck, Dorff, Hallisey, Narayanan, & Williams, 2000). Throughout history, forgiveness has been defined primarily as a philosophical, theological, and religious construct. In addition, forgiveness is a complex psychological process on both the emotional and cognitive level (Newberg, d'Aquili, Newberg, & deMarici, 2000). Within the last ten years, forgiveness has finally been discussed in the marriage and family literature (Di Blasio, 1998; Hargrave, 1994; Pollard, Anderson, Anderson, & Jennings, 1998; Ripley & Worthington, 2002). For example, family therapists have discussed forgiveness as critical in helping families with intergenerational wounds (Hargrave, 1994; DiBlasio, 1998). Furthermore, a family forgiveness scale has been developed (Pollard et al., 1998) and forgiveness has also been utilized in marital enrichment programs (Ripley & Worthington, 2002).

Empirical evidence exists indicating that forgiveness can help people manage their stress, suffering, and pain. Experimental research has shown that forgiveness can reduce feelings of revenge, anxiety, depression, anger, stress, and grief while increasing people's hope, self-esteem, and positive feelings towards offenders (Al-Mabuk, Enright, & Cardis, 1995; Coyle & Enright, 1997; Freedman & Enright, 1996; McCullough & Worthington, 1995). These studies have given forgiveness scientific credibility and increased professional interest in using forgiveness as a therapeutic and psychoeducational tool.

Most theorists believe that forgiveness is the process of giving up anger, resentment, negative judgment, and attachment to the hurt (Enright, 2001; Enright & Fitzgibbons, 2000; Luskin, 2002). Furthermore, these theorists indicate that forgiveness can allow for greater empathy and compassion for the offender, perceptual shifts, and greater contextual understanding of the offense. This change can occur when the person takes responsibility for their feelings and recognizes that old ways of resolving the hurt have not been effective. Forgiveness involves reframing the injury, changing the grievance story, and releasing pain, anger, hurt, and the need for revenge. Those who forgive can move away from blaming and accept that the injustice happened and cannot be changed. Strategies for forgiveness are developed and specific behavioral actions allow relief from the hurt. In some cases, the injured person forgives publicly by describing the positive outcomes of forgiving and their new understanding of human suffering.

## Need for Forgiveness Process Studies

Much of the recent research on forgiveness has documented that people can learn to forgive and that it can produce positive psychological outcomes. However, previous research has failed to document what happens to people during the forgiveness process. Many researchers have advocated studying the factors that facilitate the forgiveness processes (Exline & Baumeister, 2000; McCullough, Pargament, & Thoresen, 2000; Newburg et al., 2000; Pargament, McCullough, & Thoresen, 2000; Worthington, Sandage, & Berry, 2000) and indicate that process analyses are needed to determine the active ingredients of group interventions and the behavioral activity that lead to forgiveness (Newburg et al., 2000; Worthington et al., 2002). Questions have been raised about how to determine an individual's readiness to forgive (Pargament et al., 2000) and whether forgiveness produces affective and cognitive shifts, relationship improvements, and spiritual transformations (Exline & Baumeister, 2000). Significant questions have also been raised about the possible negative aspects of forgiveness (Pargament et al., 2000). Can people be hurt, revictimized, or experience regression during the process of forgiveness?

Very few, if any, published studies have assessed forgivers before the forgiveness process, during the process itself, and afterwards. Based on this lack of research, we present two studies focused on assessing the forgiveness process; first in a psychoeducational workshop over multiple time periods and then in a brief classroom intervention. Both interventions took place at a large New England University. In the workshop, participants were assessed before and during the intervention and four weeks later. The classroom intervention had a two-week follow-up. This type of assessment is crucial to understand the forgiveness process emotionally, cognitively, interpersonally, and behaviorally. Research questions addressed included: What do participants actually do or fail to do? What is the potential for forgiveness interventions to help or hurt people? What do workshop leaders and facilitators need to consider ethically ensuring that everyone is supported and protected from unintentional harm?

## STUDY 1:
## FORGIVENESS WORKSHOP

Our workshop assessment focused on four overall process areas. First, we wanted to assess preworkshop expectations, emotions, and intentions about completing workshop homework. Second, we assessed group participation and the helpfulness of leader modeling and self-disclosure. Our third process area assessed the emotional impact of the workshop and whether participants needed extra help during and after the workshop. A fourth area assessed intrapersonal, interpersonal, and behavioral activity and whether forgiveness strategies were developed.

## METHOD

### Workshop and Participants

The two-session forgiveness workshop was advertised through campus media and in university classes. Some students received extra credit for attending the workshop. Session 1 was entitled "Forgiveness Concepts and Healing Emotional Wounds"; Session 2 was entitled "Breaking Through to Forgiveness: Choosing to Take Action." There were 58 participants in Workshop Session 1; 44 returned for Workshop Session 2. Thus, the attrition rate from Session 1 to Session 2 was 24%. Participants completing both workshop sessions were primarily female (89%) and Caucasian (93%). Eighty percent of the participants were undergraduate students, 7% graduate students, 5% faculty, and 8% other adults from the community.

### Small Group Leaders

Twenty Family Studies graduate students served as small group leaders. A four-hour training session explained the forgiveness workshop process and included an experiential run-through of all of the workshop activities. A 24-page training manual was prepared to help the group leaders understand the forgiveness process and facilitate the small groups.

### Materials

Each participant was sent the book chapter "A map and tools for your journey" (Enright, 2001). This chapter focused on the process of forgiveness by describing the four phases of forgiveness and how to prepare oneself for the forgiveness process. Participants were also sent nine different definitions of forgiveness and asked to study them for common themes. A 37-page manual, "Using Forgiveness to Heal Emotional Wounds," was developed for all participants. This manual included the goals and norms of the workshop and all the forgiveness content presented in the workshop for both sessions.

## Crisis Intervention Resource Person

A PhD level psychologist was assigned the exclusive role of crisis intervention resource person. Workshop participants could meet with this person during the workshop if they were worried, upset, anxious, or in need of special assistance. Furthermore, printed information about mental health services on campus was included in all participants' workshop packets. At both the beginning and the end of each workshop, the leader discussed these potential referral sources as possible places to receive extra assistance.

## Instruments and Procedure

There were eight evaluation questionnaires specifically designed for the workshop. These questionnaires were developed by the authors to assess reactions to the workshop. They include the Preworkshop Forgiveness Needs Assessment Questionnaire, Forgiveness Reflection Assessment Sheet (Session 1), Forgiveness Phase Assessment Checklist (Session 1), Forgiveness Phase Need Assessment Checklist (Completed as Homework), Forgiveness Next Step Activity Checklist (Completed as Homework), Forgiveness Reflection Assessment Sheet 2 (Session 2), Session 1 and 2 Evaluation Questionnaires, and One Month Follow-up Questionnaire.

## FORGIVENESS WORKSHOP–SESSION 1: FORGIVENESS CONCEPTS AND HEALING EMOTIONAL WOUNDS

Table 1 shows the workshop dimensions and processes for Sessions 1 and 2. On the left are the seven dimensions of the workshop which included music, workshop lecture content, small and large group processes including the role of leader modeling and group self-disclosure, workshop checklists, and the multiple evaluations of the entire process over the eight-week period.

The workshop content was designed so that it would facilitate learning about the forgiveness process. Based on literature reviews, we selected concepts critical to understanding forgiveness and activating the

TABLE 1. Workshop Dimensions and Processes: Session 1 and Session 2

| WORKSHOP DIMENSIONS | SESSION 1 | SESSION 2 |
|---|---|---|
| MUSIC & MUSIC VIDEOS | Tango to Evora (Loreena McKennitt) (Audio) | American Tune (Simon & Garfunkel) (Video) |
| | Heart of the Matter (Don Henley) (Video) | Sounds of Silence (Simon & Garfunkel) (Video) |
| | The Old Man (John McDermott, The Irish Tenors) (Video) | |
| CONTENT–LECTURE TOPICS | Report of Needs Assessment Data<br>Positive Expectancy Setting<br>Goals and 10 Norms of the Workshop<br>Societal & Personal Context of Forgiveness<br>Wounded Person Cycle<br>What Forgiveness Is Not<br>What Forgiveness Is<br>10 Forgiveness Definitions<br>What Keeps People from Forgiving?<br>Defense Mechanisms Defined<br>Cognitive Schemas Disrupted from Pain<br>Benefits of Forgiving<br>Self-Forgiveness<br>Forgiveness Processes<br>Phases of Forgiveness<br>Campus Mental Health Resources<br>Instruction for Small Groups | Positive Expectancy Setting<br>10 Workshop Norms<br>How Do We Forgive: 21 Critical Elements?<br>Approaches to Forgiveness<br>Ways to Forgive<br>Psychological Transformation<br>Instructions for Small Groups |
| LEADER MODELING & SELF-DISCLOSURE | Workshop Leader's Disclosure (Large Group)<br>Group Leader Disclosure (Small Group) | Workshop Leader's Disclosure (Large Group)<br>Group Leader Disclosure (Small Group)<br>Workshop Members Public Disclosures |
| LARGE GROUP PROCESS | Small Group Leader Introduction<br>Psychological Resources Available | Forgiveness Phase Assessment<br>Psychological Resources Available<br>Public Disclosures About Forgiveness |
| SMALL GROUP PROCESS | 60-minute small group interaction | 90-minute small group interaction |
| CHECKLISTS USED | Forgiveness Reflection Sheet 1<br>Forgiveness Phase Assessment Checklist<br>Forgiveness Phase Needs Assessment and Next Steps Activities Checklist (Homework) | Forgiveness Reflection Sheet 2 |
| EVALUATIONS | Forgiveness Needs Assessment Questionnaire (Before Workshop)<br>Session 1 Evaluation Questionnaire | Session 2 Evaluation<br>Attrition Questionnaire<br>1 Month Follow-up Questionnaire |

healing process. The overall conceptualization of the workshop was based on five dimensions: (a) knowledge of the phases of forgiveness (Enright, 2001) and forgiveness definitions, (b) presentation of lecture content on the wounded person cycle, how human violations are internalized, and how forgiveness can set people free from their anger and pain, (c) attention to the contextual aspect of the violation and the offender's personal characteristics and motivations, (d) cognitive, emotional, and behavioral self-assessment in the context of the participant's phase of forgiveness, and, (e) strategies and action plans to implement the forgiveness process.

The workshop began with an explanation about how forgiveness is a process. The first 20 minutes were devoted to developing a collective commitment to forgiveness and group cohesion. A 3-minute reflection period with music ("Tango to Evora" by Loreena McKennitt) was used to encourage participants to think about what they wanted to accomplish in the workshop. The leader made several comments during the music, setting positive expectations for confidentiality, risk-taking, mutual support, empathy, and the potential of forgiveness as a healing force. Next, the goals of the workshop were presented as detailed in the workshop manual. The goals of the workshop were: (a) to learn the process of forgiveness in the context of the Wounded Person Cycle, (b) to derive a personal definition of forgiveness, (c) to begin the forgiveness process related to the person that hurt them, (d) to know the potential benefits of forgiving and the costs of not forgiving, (e) to discuss their forgiveness process in small and large groups at an optimal comfort level, and, (f) to evaluate the workshop. The needs assessment data were presented to communicate the collective attitudes and issues of the participants, to explain the complexity of forgiveness, and to normalize a variety of different views on forgiveness. Next, personal, national and international contexts on forgiveness were presented as well as the research documenting the positive outcomes of forgiveness.

The Wounded Person Cycle (see Figure 1) was presented as the primary context of the workshop and was used to explain the serious negative consequences of unresolved anger, resentment, rage, and pain. The seven-step cycle is the antithesis of forgiving and explains how injury and human violation negatively affect a person's psychological functioning. The first two steps of the cycle include the initial shock of the injury, along with the intense emotions of anger, rage, loss, and confusion. The shock leads to step 3, an initial quest to understand how the injury happened. In step 4, under these conditions of high emotions, distorted thinking may occur and defense mechanisms may operate to mediate intense feelings and confusing thoughts. In step 5, the wounded person may develop a grievance story, representing their attempt to understand what happened. This story may include blaming the person who wounded them and/or blaming themselves. This grievance story activates a rehearsal of the hurt, injury, and negative thoughts about the offender in step 6. These steps keep the person bonded in the negative emotions of anger and rage, thereby re-injuring him or herself and repeating the cycle all over again. One approach to disrupting the wounded person cycle was described as the breakthrough to forgiveness. Breakthroughs can occur under three conditions: (a) recognition that the injury has permanently and negatively changed the person, (b) recognition that the old strategies are not producing closure, and, (c) the consideration of healing approaches. The Wounded Person Cycle was used as a context for helping participants see the cyclical costs of harboring anger and resentment in their lives and the possibilities of forgiveness.

The forgiveness concepts were then presented as an alternative to remaining in the Wounded Person Cycle. The concepts presented included: (a) what forgiveness is and is not (Enright, 2001), (b) ten definitions of forgiveness for the participants to consider, (c) five reasons why people do not forgive, with an emphasis on how defense mechanisms and distorted cognitive schemas may inhibit processing deep pain, (d) benefits of forgiving, (e) personality characteristics of people who forgive, (f) self-forgiveness, defined as a necessary process to forgive others, and, (g) how do we forgive: 21 critical elements. Following this lecture, Don Henley's "Heart of the Matter" music video was played to emphasize the difficulty and complexity of forgiving others and ourselves.

After a short break, the small group leaders introduced themselves by stating their positive expectations for the workshop process. Following this second context-setting activity, the primary leader of the workshop modeled self-disclosure by discussing the process of forgiving his father. This included describing the family dynamics of the hurtful events and how they affected his life. The moving music video, "The Old Man" by the Irish Tenors, was played to emphasize what the workshop leader had lost by having a broken relationship with his father. The purpose of this self-disclosure was to set the stage for the participants to begin their own forgiveness in the small groups.

Participants were prepared for their small group experience by filling out the *Forgiveness Reflection Sheet 1*. The workshop then broke into small groups to discuss the *Forgiveness Reflection Sheet* for one hour.

FIGURE 1. The Wounded Person Cycle

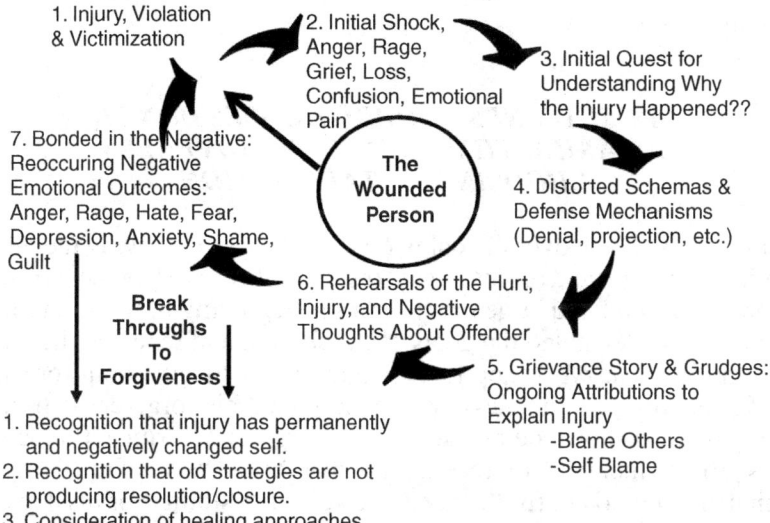

After the group leaders established the small group norms, each leader disclosed their personal information on their *Forgiveness Reflection Sheet*, as a way of modeling self-disclosure in the group process. Each member of the group was asked to participate at their optimal comfort level. One group leader took notes on the group's collective disclosures. After returning to the large group, the small group leaders gave a short summary of their group's work.

Following this, the workshop participants were given a short lecture on the phases of the forgiveness process using Enright's Phases and Units of Forgiving (Enright, 2001; Enright & Fitzgibbons, 2000). Students were asked to fill out the *Forgiveness Phase Assessment Checklist* that assessed the four phases using specific behavioral descriptions. They were asked to select one of the four phases that best captured their current place in the forgiveness process. Participants were then given homework assignments to complete between sessions including the *Forgiveness Phase Need Assessment Checklist* and the *Forgiveness Next Steps Activity Checklist*. Participants were encouraged to consider implementing forgiveness process activities over the next week. The session ended with the *Session 1 Evaluation Questionnaire*. Participants were reminded that they could contact their small group leader or the workshop leader if they needed special assistance over the next week. After the workshop, small group leaders were debriefed in a 45-minute session.

## FORGIVENESS WORKSHOP–SESSION 2: BREAKING THROUGH TO FORGIVENESS– CHOOSING TO TAKE ACTION

In Session 2, the overall goal was to spend time reviewing the homework assignment and discussing next steps with the forgiveness process in both the small and large groups. At the beginning of the session, the workshop leader stated the goals of the session and repeated the workshop norms. The workshop leader continued his story about forgiving his father from the first session. He explained his forgiveness process using the workshop lecture "How do we forgive: 21 Critical Elements." This process included: (a) recognizing that the old ways of resolving the pain had not worked, (b) the need to take responsibility for his negative feelings, (c) developing a new contextual and compassionate perspective on his father that allowed him to reframe the injury, have empathy for his father, and stop the blaming, (d) creating a perceptual shift in how he defined the father-son relationship, (e) changing the old grievance story, (f) recognizing that his own capacity for fathering would be affected if he did not continue the process of forgiving his father, and, (g) discovering meaning in his suffering and the positive outcomes of forgiving. This was followed by two brief lectures on approaches to forgiveness and ways to implement forgiveness.

Next, the workshop participants filled out *Forgiveness Reflection Sheet 2*. After completing this exercise in the large group, the small groups convened for 90 minutes. The small group leaders restated the group norms and disclosed their own forgiveness process over the week as well as their next steps. The final activity of the workshop was the invitation for workshop participants to publicly disclose their forgiveness process, by stating what they had done and what they plan to do in the future. The large group leader facilitated this series of disclosures until the *Session 2 Evaluation Questionnaire* was completed. The workshop closed with two music videos–"American Tune" and "Sounds of Silence" by Simon and Garfunkel. Participants were reminded that the workshop leaders were available to them after the workshop. Following the workshop, the group leaders were debriefed in a 30-minute session.

## RESULTS

A total of 108 process questions were asked of each participant over an eight-week period. All the questionnaire items were analyzed by clustering them into the five forgiveness process areas. Four questionnaires assessed participants' forgiveness before, during, and after the workshops. All questionnaires used a Likert scale ranging from 4 (Strongly Agree) to 1 (Strongly Disagree). The data were calculated by adding the Strongly Agree (4) and Agree (3) together for each questionnaire item to derive a composite agreement number. All frequency data were transformed to percentages to derive a total percent agreement for each item. Return rates for all questionnaires ranged between 77 and 91%.

### Preworkshop Expectancies, Emotions, and Intentions to Complete Homework

The needs assessment data indicated that the registrants had positive expectancies about attending the forgiveness workshop and positive emotions about the forgiveness process. Over 90% of the participants believed that forgiveness could improve their lives and promote personal growth. Over 80% indicated willingness to put extra effort into the workshop and participate in the small groups. Willingness to take personal risks in the workshop was reported by over 60% of the participants. On an emotional level, 70% reported anger at a person they wanted to forgive and 56% reported wanting to let go of this anger during the workshop. Forty percent of those who attended reported that their past attempts at forgiving had not worked and just under 30% enrolled in the workshop because they failed to forgive in the past. One quarter of the participants expected that the workshop would be difficult for them. Fifteen percent worried about taking the workshop and 62% reported needing to forgive themselves before forgiving others. Over 30% of those who attended indicated that they might need extra help during the workshop and 90% understood that extra help was available to them during and after the workshop.

There were four assessments of workshop members' intentions to participate and complete the workshop homework assignments. The purpose of this was to better understand participants' motivation levels and the degree to which they followed through by completing the homework assignments. Before the workshop, 80% of the participants reported they would do the forgiveness reading and 90% reported they would review the definitions of forgiveness. At the end of the first session, over 85% of the participants reported they wanted to discuss their forgiveness processes and next steps in session 2. Furthermore, over 90% agreed to spend an hour on the next step homework assignment. During the second session, 70% actually reported doing the assignment.

## Group Participation, Satisfaction and Helpfulness of Leader Modeling and Disclosure

The small groups were reported to be helpful by 87% of the participants in session 1 and 83% for session 2. In both sessions, over 80% of the workshop members reported participating in their small groups and after session two, 93% reported talking about their specific forgiveness process. During the final session, 73% of the participants reported making a public statement about their forgiveness process in either the small or large group.

One of the major workshop interventions was the use of group leaders' self-disclosure and modeling of their forgiveness process. In both sessions, over 90% of the participants reported that the workshop leader's self-disclosure about forgiving his father made them more comfortable with their own forgiveness processes. Eighty-nine percent of the participants in session 1 and 95% of the participants in session 2 reported that the small group leaders' self-disclosures about their forgiveness processes helped them open up. Furthermore, 98% of the participants reported that peer disclosures helped facilitate their forgiveness process.

## Emotional Impact of the Workshop and Need for Extra Help

Many feelings were reported by 97% of the participants immediately after session 1 and 11% reported the workshop was too intense for them. Between sessions 1 and 2, 32% experienced pain when working with their forgiveness process and 25% reported emotional turmoil. Immediately after session 2, 88% reported many feelings but only 5% reported the workshop was too intense. There was also emotional comfort and release reported. After session 2, 87% of workshop members reported being more comfortable with their emotional pain, 72% reported letting go of some their anger at the person who had hurt them, and 35% reported crying during or after the workshop. Whether the emotionality of the forgiveness workshop continued over time was assessed through the one-month follow-up. Since the end of the workshop, 71% of the participants reported letting go of anger at the person who hurt them, while 60% were still experiencing pain from the workshop. Fifty-four percent reported experiencing continuous emotions about the forgiveness process, and 42% reported crying from their forgiveness process one month after the workshop.

Before the workshop, the need for extra help during the workshop process was expressed by 31% of the participants and another 29% were unsure about the need for additional help. After session 1, the reported need for extra help jumped to 56%. After session 2, the need for extra help decreased to 35%. Even with this decrease, 46% of participants planned to seek help, 38% reported a need for an additional forgiveness session, and 35% reported a need for counseling to continue their forgiveness process.

## Intrapersonal, Interpersonal, and Behavioral Activity and Forgiveness Strategies

Intrapersonal forgiveness was operationally defined as the internal thinking processes of the participants before, during, and after the workshop. At the end of session 1, 74% of the participants had a lot of questions about their personal forgiveness process and 54% were able to decide which phase of forgiveness they were in. By the end of session 2, 73% were able to determine their exact forgiveness phase. In between sessions 1 and 2, 88% of the workshop members had forgiveness on their mind and 80% reported thinking about the person who had hurt them in terms of their motivations and current life situation. At the end of workshop session 2, 90% of the participants reported a greater clarification of their forgiveness definition, 87% reported being more comfortable with their emotional pain, and 83% found more meaning in their suffering. Furthermore, at the end of the workshop, 64% reported a perceptual shift in how they viewed the person they were forgiving and 37% had changed their grievance story about the offender. Finally, over 80% of the participants reported making progress with their forgiveness process at the end of the workshop and everyone reported they were glad they had taken the program.

The one-month follow-up indicated that internal cognitive processing continued after the workshop ended. Eighty-nine percent of the participants had ongoing thinking about forgiveness and over 90% thought about, heard, or observed something related to forgiveness. Since the workshop, 83% of the participants had thoughts about other people's small group disclosures. Sixty-eight percent thought about communicating with the person who had hurt them, 58% thought about their grievance story related to their personal hurt, and over 60% reported a perceptual shift with the person who hurt them. Sixty percent reported still working on forgiving themselves.

The results also indicate behavioral activity between sessions and after the workshop. Over 70% of the participants reported working on their forgiveness process between sessions. Furthermore, between sessions, 70% spoke to another person about their forgiveness process. One month later, behavioral action since the workshop was also evident. Over 80% of the workshop members had initiated a conversation with another person about forgiveness and 68% initiated a conversation about their own personal forgiveness processes. Seventy-one percent of the participants reported taking some action with their forgiveness processes, 68% reported making progress with forgiveness, and just slightly fewer than 50% had spoken to or had communication with the person they wanted to forgive.

How well the forgiveness workshop taught forgiveness strategies and next steps were assessed after session 2 and one month later. After session 2, 86% of the participants reported that because of the workshop, they had strategies for forgiveness, but 58% reported a need for additional strategies to actualize their forgiveness. One month later, 74% reported using their forgiveness strategies, but 40% still reported confusion about next steps in their forgiveness processes.

## STUDY 2:
## CLASSROOM FORGIVENESS INTERVENTION

Over the last eight years, a significantly shortened version of the forgiveness workshop has been used in the University of Connecticut Family Studies' undergraduate course "Introduction to Counseling." The shortened classroom version included all of the lecture material on what forgiveness is, how to do it, much of the media, and the instructor's disclosure and modeling of forgiving his father. The students were 85% female, predominately white, and in their early twenties.

Students were asked to fill out *Forgiveness Reflection Sheet 1*. This exercise invited them to choose someone they need to forgive. The students described in writing their feelings for the person they wanted to forgive. The students answered the question: Can I forgive this person or not? They then wrote out their reasons for forgiving or deciding not to forgive. The classroom intervention occurred over a 10-day period in three, 90-minute classes. A two-week follow-up evaluation was conducted with the students (n = 49) using the same questionnaire items from the workshop.

## RESULTS

The results indicate that a short forgiveness intervention can be implemented in a classroom setting and have an emotional and behavioral impact. Eighty-two percent of the students indicated that they had made some progress with their forgiveness process over the two-week period. Sixty-seven percent indicated that they had used some of the forgiveness strategies and 45% indicated they had spoken to another person about their own forgiveness process. Sixty-seven percent disclosed they had a perceptual shift with the person who hurt them. In terms of behavioral activity of the students, 53% reported having communicated with the person they wanted to forgive.

The classroom intervention was also an emotional experience for students. Sixty-seven percent of the students indicated an emotional reaction to their forgiveness process over the two-week period and 63% reported pain from working with their forgiveness process. Thirty-three percent of the students reported crying while experiencing the forgiveness process and 82% reported letting go of their anger at the person who had hurt them. Only 5% of the students reported that the forgiveness classes were too intense. Ninety-nine percent indicated that the professor's disclosure about forgiving his father helped them with their own forgiveness processes. Over 50% of the students reported they were still confused on how to proceed with their forgiveness process. Over 60% of the students had unanswered questions about their forgiveness process. Forty-three percent reported that they needed extra help with their forgiveness process and 67% indicated they would like to attend a more expansive forgiveness workshop. Finally, 98% of students recommended that the forgiveness intervention be continued in future classes.

## DISCUSSION

The process evaluation indicates that the participants were positively affected by the forgiveness workshop and classroom interventions in multiple ways over the two- and eight-week periods. The results also suggest that cognitive, affective, and behavioral shifts can occur from brief forgiveness interventions. The implications and limitations of the data, the need for future research, and our recommendations for improving future forgiveness interventions are summarized below.

The data indicate that many of the participants had positive expectancies about the workshop and were willing to prepare for the process. The workshop norms and homework assignments were effective in orienting most of the participants to the positive power of forgiveness. Not all participants were fully engaged in the workshop. Twenty percent of the participants did not complete the preworkshop homework and 30% failed to complete the between session assignment. Additional strategies are needed to ensure that out-of-workshop assignments are completed. We recommend contracting with participants about completing homework assignments or conducting screening interviews to determine the appropriateness of forgiveness interventions for unmotivated or fragile participants. This kind of screening also may decrease the amount of attrition from the workshop.

The data also indicate that the workshop was emotionally and cognitively charged for many of the participants. Nearly half of the participants either worried about taking the workshop or indicated that it would be difficult for them. Many of the participants reported highly emotional experiences during the workshop and in the classroom intervention. We recommend that future workshops provide more opportunities for participants to receive personal assistance with these intense emotions. We also strongly recommend that future workshops continue our practice of disseminating information about mental health resources on campus and in the community. Furthermore, the data strongly support having a crisis intervention resource professional available during any large-scale educational workshop on sensitive topics. During our workshop, this resource person was busy with participants who were fragile and having trouble coping with their intense feelings. This crisis professional helped us avert potential "fallout" from the workshop and overall disruption of the workshop process.

One of the strongest findings of the workshop was that the group process and leader modeling through self-disclosure sections were very effective parts of the intervention. Over 80% of the participants spoke in the groups and reported the groups were helpful to them and over 90% of the participants indicated that the personal disclosures of the group leaders helped them open up and become more comfortable. Based on these results, the continued use of groups and leader self-disclosure and modeling during forgiveness workshops is strongly recommended.

The evaluation of results from both the workshop and classroom intervention indicated that many of the participants learned strategies of forgiveness, but they were also left with confusion and unanswered questions about the next steps. We recommend that increased time be devoted to the pragmatics and strategies of forgiveness using case studies and concrete examples. For example, over 60% of the participants reported needing to do self-forgiveness both before and after the workshop. Some forgiveness theorists suggest that self-forgiveness is an important process in forgiving others (Casarjian, 1992; Luskin, 2002). Thus, future interventions should spend more time on self-forgiveness due to its potential impact on the healing process.

Many of our recommendations could be reduced to a single insight: The workshop and classroom intervention needed to be longer in duration to respond to the unanswered questions, need for strategies, and extra help. There is little doubt that a longer workshop would have made the process even more effective. More small and large group time for unstructured talking about the complexities of forgiveness may be needed for interventions to have their maximum effect.

The results revealed that many participants were activated cognitively, emotionally, and behaviorally. Over 60% of the participants in both interventions let go of their anger at the person who hurt them, experienced emotional discharge and perceptual shifts, and felt pain from the workshop. These results were consistent immediately after the workshop and one month later as well as with the classroom program. Additionally, much intrapersonal and interpersonal activity was reported, with 50% of the participants actually confronting or communicating with their offender.

Limitations to our process evaluation need to be considered when interpreting the data. The results may have been influenced by using college students who received course credit for their participation. Furthermore, the results are mainly generalized to undergraduate female students. Future forgiveness workshops should examine whether men, older adults, and racially and ethnically diverse samples react to being taught forgiveness skills in similar or different ways. Also, only non-standardized self-report questionnaires were used in the evaluation. We recommend more complex designs when assessing future forgiveness interventions using standardized measures of change, control groups, and more elaborate process designs.

In summary, the forgiveness workshop was a moving experience for the participants and the group facilitators. We witnessed the power of forgiveness and observed participants liberating themselves from their pain and emotional wounds. We observed many participants break out of the Wounded Person Cycle (see Figure 1) by using forgiveness concepts and processes. We observed participants engage in self-disclosure about forgiveness in both large and small groups. Many of the participants used their emerging insights outside the workshop. We advocate further experimentation and evaluation of psychoeducational interventions that teach people how to forgive. Our interventions have convinced us that people can learn forgiveness skills and heal their emotional wounds. Many of people's wounds occur during family and marital interactions. Therefore, we recommend that family life educators and other professionals become more active in promoting forgiveness with students, families, and the larger society.

## REFERENCES

Al-Mabuk, R.H., Enright, R.D., & Cardis, P.A. (1995). Forgiveness education with parentally love deprived late adolescents. *Journal of Moral Education, 24*, 427-444.

Casarjian, R. (1992). *Forgiveness: A bold choice for a peaceful heart.* New York: Bantam.

Coyle, C.T. & Enright, R.D. (1997). Forgiveness intervention with post abortion men. *Journal of Consulting and Clinical Psychology, 65*, 1042-1046.

DiBlasio, F.A. (1998). The use of a decision-based forgiveness intervention within intergenerational family therapy. *Journal of Family Therapy, 20*, 79-94.

Enright, R.D. (2001). *Forgiveness is a choice: A step-by-step process for resolving anger and restoring hope.* Washington, D.C.: American Psychological Association.

Enright, R.D. & Fitzgibbons, R.P. (2000). *Helping clients forgive: An empirical guide for resolving anger and restoring hope.* Washington, D.C.: American Psychological Association.

Exline, J.J. & Baumeister, R.F. (2000). Expressing forgiveness and repentance: Benefits and barriers. In M.E. McCullough, K.I. Pargament, & C.E. Thoresen (Eds.), *Forgiveness: Theory, research and practice* (pp. 133-155). New York: Guilford Press.

Freedman, S.R. & Enright, R.D. (1996). Forgiveness as in intervention goal with incest survivors. *Journal of Consulting and Clinical Psychology, 64*, 983-992.

Hargrave, T.D. (1994). *Families and forgiveness: Healing wounds in the intergenerational family.* New York: Brunner/Mazel.

Luskin, F. (2002). *Forgive for good.* San Francisco, CA: Harper Collins.

McCullough, M.E., Pargament, K.I., & Thoresen, C.E. (Eds.). (2000). *Forgiveness: Theory, research, and practice.* New York: Guilford Press.

McCullough, M.E. & Worthington, E.L. (1995). Promoting forgiveness: A comparison of two brief psychoeducational group interventions with waiting list control. *Counseling and Values, 40*, 55-68.

Newberg, A.B., d'Aquili, E.G., Newberg, S.K., & deMarici, V. (2000). The neuropsychological correlates of forgiveness. In M.E. McCullough, K.I. Pargament, &

C.E. Thoresen (Eds.), *Forgiveness: Theory, research and practice* (pp. 91-110). New York: Guilford Press.

Pargament, K.I., McCullough, M.E., & Thoresen, C.E. (2000). The frontier of forgiveness: Seven directions for psychological study and practice. In M.E. McCullough, K.I. Pargament, & C.E. Thoresen (Eds.), *Forgiveness: Theory, research and practice* (pp. 229-319). New York: Guilford Press.

Pollard, M.W., Anderson, R.A., Anderson, W.T., & Jennings, G. (1998). The development of a family forgiveness scale. *Journal of Family Therapy, 20*, 95-109.

Ripley, J.S. & Worthington, E.L. (2002). Hope-focused and forgiveness-based group interventions to promote marital enrichment. *Journal of Counseling & Development, 80*, 452-463.

Rye, M.S., Pargament, K.I., Ali, M.A., Beck, G.L., Dorff, E.N., Hallisey, C., Narayanan, V., & Williams, J.G. (2000). Religious perspectives on forgiveness. In M.E. McCullough, K.I. Pargament, & C.E. Thoresen (Eds.), *Forgiveness: Theory, research, and practice* (pp. 17-40). New York: Guilford.

Worthington, E.L., Sandage, S.J., & Berry, J.W. (2002). Group interventions to promote forgiveness: What researchers and clinicians ought to know. In M.E. McCullough, K.I. Pargament, & C.E. Thoresen (Eds.), *Forgiveness: Theory, research and practice* (pp. 228-253). New York: Guilford Press.

# The Impact of Service-Learning on Student Development: Students' Reflections in a Family Diversity Course

Michelle L. Toews
Jennifer M. Cerny

**ABSTRACT.** The purpose of this study was to gain a better understanding of the personal, professional, interpersonal, social, and academic development of students who complete a 15-hour service-learning assignment as part of the requirements for a family diversity course. A content analysis of 36 students' reflection papers revealed that service-learning was extremely beneficial, even when the experience was brief. Numerous valuable lessons were learned by the students about themselves and their future careers. Specifically, they became more accepting of others, and they realized the importance of service to one's community. In addition, they were able to process and synthesize the information they learned in the classroom by experiencing the course content in a real-world setting. *[Article copies available for a fee from The Haworth Document Delivery Service: 1-800-HAWORTH. E-mail address: <docdelivery@haworthpress.com> Website: <http://www.HaworthPress.com> © 2005 by The Haworth Press, Inc. All rights reserved.]*

---

Michelle L. Toews and Jennifer M. Cerny are affiliated with Texas State University-San Marcos.

Address correspondence to: Michelle L. Toews, Texas State University-San Marcos, Department of Family and Consumer Sciences, 601 University Drive, San Marcos, TX 78666 (E-mail: mt15@txstate.edu).

**KEYWORDS.** Service-learning, family science, college students, student development, family diversity course

## INTRODUCTION

At universities across the country, there is a growing interest in integrating service-learning into the curriculum. For those unfamiliar with service-learning, it is a form of experiential education where students learn the course content while applying their knowledge in the community (Eby, 2001; Martin, 2001). Service-learning is particularly effective when incorporated into family science courses (see Eby, 2001 & Galbraith, 2002 for a complete overview). Without it, students may "be limited in their ability to really comprehend and appreciate the theoretical material because of a lack of practical experience working with individuals or families" (Galbraith, 2002, p. 364). Furthermore, by integrating service-learning and classroom instruction, family science professors are not only enhancing the students' understanding of course content and social issues, but are also preparing their students to work in the family science field by helping them develop tolerance, empathy, and a sense of civic responsibility (Astin & Sax, 1998; Burnett, Hamel, & Long, 2004; Eyler & Giles, 1999; Sedlak, Doheny, Panthofer, & Anaya, 2003). In addition, other positive outcomes of service-learning have been found and can typically be grouped into five categories of development: personal, professional, interpersonal, social, and academic.

### *Personal Development*

In previous studies, one of the most frequently reported outcomes of service-learning was increased self-efficacy among students (Astin, Vogelgesang, Ikeda, & Yee, 2001; Giles & Eyler, 1994; Morgan & Streb, 2001; Sedlak et al., 2003). In fact, Giles and Eyler (1994) noted that not only was increased self-efficacy a benefit of service-learning, it was also a predictor of whether individuals would become involved. Furthermore, the students reported a belief that they could make a difference in the communities they served. This is a significant finding in that a resistant attitude toward service-learning may prevent students from gaining the maximum benefit from the experience.

Service-learning also fosters students' personal development by putting them in situations they have not been exposed to previously. As a result, students discovered personal strengths they were unaware of prior to this experience (Walker, Blankemeyer, Richardson, & Kraynak, 2003). In addition, Sedlak and colleagues (2003) found that service-learning helped students evaluate their own values and beliefs. Martin (2001) also found that students' personal values were questioned during their service-learning experiences, which enhanced self-awareness (Eyler & Giles, 1999; Hamilton & Fenzel, 1988) and clarified personal values and beliefs (Astin et al., 2001).

## Professional Development

Previous researchers also have found that service-learning helps prepare students for their future careers. For example, students report increased leadership skills (Astin et al., 2001; Eyler & Giles, 1999), enhanced communication skills, professional growth (Sedlak et al., 2003), and increased confidence to proceed with their chosen careers (Walker et al., 2003; Yates & Youniss, 1996). Morgan (1997-1998) found that high school students who participated in service-learning developed more confidence speaking in public, a useful skill for multiple professions. Additionally, researchers found that service-learning allows students to reassess their future career plans (Dudderar & Stover, 2003; Walker et al., 2003). Not surprisingly, after participating in service learning activities, some students decided not to pursue a career in their initial field of interest, while others reaffirmed their decisions.

## Interpersonal Development

Previous researchers found a plethora of positive results regarding students' interpersonal development through service-learning, but two in particular stand out. One, it was found that the experience resulted in a better understanding of other cultures (Astin et al., 2001; Eyler & Giles, 1999; Giles & Eyler, 1994; Yates & Youniss, 1996), consequently producing an increased tolerance of individuals different from themselves (Eyler & Giles, 1999; Morgan & Streb, 2001; Sedlak et al., 2003). And two, many became more appreciative of the diversity of cultures they worked with during their service-learning experience (Eyler & Giles, 1999; Sedlak et al., 2003).

Along these same lines, Eyler and Giles (1999) found that college students who participated in a one credit "community service laboratory" reported greater ability to work with others and held fewer negative stereotypes about those with whom they worked. In a similar study, Giles and Eyler (1994) found that college students were less likely to blame social clients for their situations. In addition, after participating in their service-learning experience, college students held a more positive image of the people with whom they worked and developed a greater sense of concern for others (Scales, Blyth, Berkas, & Kielsmeier, 2000; Sedlak et al., 2003).

## Social Development

With respect to social development, previous research concluded that participation in service-learning projects significantly increased social responsibility (Astin & Sax, 1998; Conrad & Hedin, 1982; Giles & Eyler, 1994; Markus, Arbor, Howard, & King, 1993; Scales et al., 2000; Sedlak et al., 2003). Social responsibility generally refers to reducing stereotypes, developing empathetic understanding, and gaining a stronger sense of opportunity and achievement (Giles & Eyler, 1994). Not only did service learning experiences enable students to become directly involved in community service, it often continued in the form of volunteer work the following semester (Astin et al., 2001; Giles & Eyler, 1994). Additionally, most students who participated in service-learning felt more connected to their communities (Eyler & Giles, 1999; Karasik & Berke, 2001).

## Academic Development

Numerous studies found that students enrolled in service-learning courses displayed a significant improvement in academic performance, overall grade point average, and attendance (Astin et al., 2001; Morgan, 1997-1998; Stukas, Clary, & Snyder, 1999). Crowner (1992) concluded that students enjoyed service-learning assignments and reported learning more through practical experience than from the traditional class format. As a general rule, most studies found that incorporating service-learning into a course enhances the understanding of the core content and gives students a greater ability to apply classroom knowledge to real life situations (Eyler & Giles, 1999; Markus et al., 1993). Additionally, service-learning helped students get more out of the classroom experience. Morgan (1997-1998), for example, found that students enrolled in a course requiring service-learning were not only more prepared for class, but were more likely to discuss course content outside of the classroom. Other studies also have shown that service-learning makes students more interested and engaged in the classroom (Astin et al., 2001; Scales et al., 2000).

Based on this review of the literature, it is clear that service-learning is associated with positive student outcomes such as increased self-efficacy, greater self-knowledge, increased tolerance of differences, greater sense of civic and social responsibility, and improved academic outcomes (e.g., Astin et al., 2001; Eyler & Giles, 1999; Morgan & Streb, 2001; Scales et al., 2000; Sedlak et al., 2003). However, most researchers have not examined the potential benefits of brief service-learning experiences (Giles & Eyler, 1994) as opposed to service-learning courses or a service-learning internship or practicum. The goal of this study, therefore, was to gain a better understanding of the personal, professional, interpersonal, social, and academic development of students who complete a brief (15 hour) service-learning assignment.

## METHODOLOGY

### Participants and Procedures

The sample consisted of 36 family and consumer sciences majors, all females, enrolled in a family diversity class. As part of the requirements for this upper-level family and child development course, each student was required to work directly with families and/or children for a minimum of 15 unpaid hours at a site pre-approved by their professor. It was suggested that the required hours be distributed over the course of the semester (i.e., 1-2 hours per week); however, flexibility in scheduling was granted with permission from both the professor and the on-site supervisor.

In addition, the students were required to write a paper (7-10 pages) at the end of the semester reflecting on what they learned about themselves and others and to what degree the service learning assignment related to course content (Galbraith, 2002; Terry & Bohnenberger, 2003). Specifically, the students were instructed to provide a brief description of their service-learning site and duties (10 points), as well as reflect on their experiences by asking themselves the following questions: (a) What did I learn about myself through this experience? What realizations, insights, or lessons did I learn? (15 points); (b) Was there a moment of failure, success, indecision, doubt, humor, frustration, happiness, sadness, etc.? What was my greatest accomplishment? What was my biggest challenge? (15 points); (c) Has this experience challenged stereotypes or prejudices I have? If so, how? Will this experience change the way I act or think in the future? (15 points); (d) In what ways could I apply the lessons I have learned to other areas of my life? (10 points); and (e) How did this experience compliment or contrast with what I learned in class? Has learning through experience taught me more, less, or the same as the class? In what ways? (15 points). The paper was graded based on grammar, spelling, punctuation, and other components of good writing (10 points), as well as the breadth and depth of the students' reflections.

*Data Analysis*

After securing permission from the students to use their papers in this qualitative study, a manual content analysis was conducted by three independent coders to assure a more reliable and valid analysis (Berg, 1998). Inductively, reoccurring themes within and commonalities among the students' responses were identified and sorted based on similar themes (Berg, 1998). To represent these themes and commonalities, initial coding categories (i.e., broad categories such as what the students learned about themselves, others, and the connection between course content and service-learning) were developed. Next, the data were examined deductively to identify more specific themes such as personal, professional, interpersonal, social, and academic development. Lastly, the primary coder examined the identified themes to determine if the findings were consistent among the coders. Any inconsistencies were discussed by the coders until consensus was reached.

## FINDINGS

The goal of this study was to explore and describe the benefits of integrating a brief service-learning assignment into a family diversity course and to understand, from the students' point of view, how service-learning enhanced their personal, professional, interpersonal, social, and academic development. In this section, we present the students' descriptions of the ways in which service-learning impacted their development. In addition, Table 1 presents an overview of how many students commented on each theme and the number of times each theme was mentioned within the students' reflections.

*Personal Development*

A commonly reported theme among 36% of the students was an increased sense of self-efficacy. Participating in this brief service-learn-

TABLE 1. Results of Analysis by Themes

| Area of development and sub-themes | No. of times mentioned | No. of students who mentioned |
|---|---|---|
| Personal | 43 | 27 |
| Self-efficacy | 15 | 13 |
| Patience | 22 | 18 |
| Time management | 6 | 6 |
| Professional | 9 | 9 |
| Confidence | 2 | 2 |
| Reaffirmed future career | 5 | 5 |
| Deterred away from chosen career | 3 | 3 |
| Interpersonal | 61 | 28 |
| Increased tolerance of diversity | 36 | 23 |
| Greater social awareness | 14 | 11 |
| Importance of listening | 11 | 9 |
| Social | 15 | 9 |
| Importance of community service | 11 | 9 |
| Committed to future service | 4 | 4 |
| Academic | 35 | 28 |
| Increased understanding of course content | 23 | 22 |
| Learned more through experience | 12 | 12 |

ing experience gave students confidence in their ability to make a difference in a person's life. One student summarized her experience by saying, "I felt my self-esteem rise. Realizing that I can have that big of an impact on children's lives is the most valuable lesson I believe I can ever learn." After working in an after-school program at a local housing authority, one student reported, "I feel that this experience has really helped me with my self-esteem because I know that I can make a difference in situations as long as I speak up and act on my feelings." Another student reported, "I feel my greatest accomplishment and my greatest challenge was working with the kids on a one-on-one basis. I don't feel comfortable taking care of other people's kids so to volunteer with this program [a day-care for children of teen parents] was a big step for me. I think I was able to see I wasn't as bad with children as I thought."

Even students who were not "expecting much out of the service-learning requirement" for the course felt as though it was a valuable experience. For example, one student who worked in a mentoring program stated that service-learning "was not what I expected it to be at all. I honestly went in with the intent of working my 15 hours and then writing a paper, all for a grade–not even thinking twice that I could possibly get something out of this experience. I just kept thinking, what could I do to help other people? I soon realized that I could do a lot to help." She also commented, "The experience was well worth it; knowing that I was making a difference made me feel like there was nothing that I could not do."

There were a few instances when the students' frustrations created a lack of self-efficacy. One student reported, "I definitely had moments of doubts. There were times I felt like my presence served no purpose. I doubted whether I was really making a difference. I also had moments where I felt like a failure when I was interacting with [the child]." Another student commented, "There were a few times when I felt frustration and then failure. This was when the kids didn't want to cooperate because they weren't interested in the lesson." However, many times the situation eventually turned around to be a positive experience: "There were several times throughout the semester when I felt extremely frustrated because I felt like I was making no progress in connecting with the kids. Some nights I came home so discouraged because it seemed the entire evening had merely been crowd control. However, as the semester progressed, I was blessed to get to see some of the ways that lives were being changed."

Another theme reported by 50 percent of the students was improved patience when working with other individuals, particularly children. As expressed by one student: "From this, I have become more patient with children, even though I already considered myself fairly patient." A student working with preschool-aged children in a child development center remarked, "Having gone through this experience at the center has definitely taught me patience, understanding, and has made me stronger as an individual." Lastly, one student felt that the patience she learned through her experience working as a parent liaison for a play therapist was something she could utilize in both her career and her personal life.

Close to 20 percent of the students also felt that adding service-learning hours to their already busy schedules helped them develop better time management and organization skills. This theme was clearly demonstrated by one student's statement, "I have also learned better time management skills by having to go to class, then volunteering, and then straight to work for the rest of the day." As one student briefly explains, "I quickly had to learn to manage my time better." Another felt it helped her become more organized.

## Professional Development

In addition to their personal development and increased sense of self-efficacy, 25 percent of the students also reported themes related to their professional development, even though this was not directly asked. For example, two students reported more competence in their abilities as family professionals. One student stated she now "felt competent in working with not only children, but with their families as well." Another student acknowledged, "This experience has really given me the confidence that I can be successful with my degree."

A second theme associated with professional development concerned the students' evaluation of their future career choices. For some students (n = 5), their service-learning experience reaffirmed their aspirations of pursuing a career working with families. As one student stated, "I learned that there is not a doubt in my mind that I want to pursue this career with all my heart." Another student shared similar sentiments: "I learned my future career will be dedicated to parents with at-risk children or at-risk families in general." One student who worked with at-risk children believed her experience truly reaffirmed her decision to pursue a career in child psychology.

After participating in this brief service-learning experience, on the other hand, three students decided against working in the family and child development field. As one student stated, "I do not feel that I am emotionally able to do this type of work." Another expressed relief: "I am so thankful for the opportunity to work in this setting and realize it was not meant for me."

## Interpersonal Development

One of the most beneficial aspects of service-learning also coincided with the primary objective of the course: an increased appreciation for diversity within and among families. Two-thirds of the students reported they were more aware of previous stereotypes they held and had become more tolerant of diverse family forms and cultures. For one student, the experience taught her "how to effectively work with many different children from many different socio-ethnic groups." Working with diverse families in a program aimed at improving parent-child communication helped another student become more tolerant of others.

Similarly, students became aware of previous stereotypes they held and were able to view various situations and individuals with a more open mind. Reflecting on her service-learning experience working with a small group of youth from a local church, one student said, "One of the most important life lessons I have learned through this experience is not to 'label' or assume I have people figured out before getting to know them." Working with the infants in a high school program for adolescent parents taught one student "not to judge other individuals or families before knowing their situation." Another student mentoring children from an after-school program in a government housing complex felt her experience taught her to open her eyes to other people's perspectives. After volunteering at a Head Start program, one student stated, "I learned not to be so judgmental of people because you never know where they are coming from."

This same student reported, "I now know the hardships they went through and what they had to endure as children. I can now relate in some way to these children and how they live." Many other students also reported an increased sense of empathy for the families they encountered. For example, one student felt more sympathy for working single moms because she saw how hard it was for them to juggle everything in their lives. Another student felt her experience working with at-risk children drastically changed the way she previously viewed welfare recipients: "I thought that they may be lazy or that they did not try. I realized that this is not necessarily true. Most of the parents do try very hard to support their children. They do try to provide them with the best things that they can. I also saw them try to be involved in their child's life and wanting to be more. Because some of my stereotypes have changed, in the future I may not look at welfare so harshly."

Additionally, one-third of the students reported they were more aware of the harsh realities many families face. Students' comments demonstrating this theme included: "I realized I have lived a sheltered life and there is a lot of heartache in the world of which I was not aware. I'm glad I'm more aware because now I can understand more of what they are going through. This experience has opened my eyes to see that I have been living in my own little bubble for a long time. It is easy to ignore things if you don't know that things, such as domestic violence, are really going on around you. I don't want to ignore them anymore."

As the previous quote indicates, this experience made students realize that these issues were affecting families in their communities. After working with a group of first-graders through a church program in a very small town, one student explained, "One of the benefits of this experience has been that it allowed me to see that there are hurting children in my community. I do not have to go to inner city New York to find children who have been touched by abuse, neglect, or the emotional stress that can accompany families of divorce." One student had the opportunity to volunteer at a residential facility for children with criminal backgrounds. When reflecting on her experience, she stated, "I came to understand the reality of troubled families. Many times I think we can overlook the reality of troubled families when we are not forced to encounter it everyday."

Lastly, 25 percent of the students reported realizing how important it was to listen to others. After spending her service-learning hours working with a play therapist, one particular student stated, "Through this experience I have discovered the value of listening. Children have a lot to say, and a lot that needs to be heard. Simply listening to a child can prevent many behavior problems." Another student, who had worked with a group of children on communication skills, anger management, and coping strategies, reiterated this fact: "I also learned that children just want to be listened to. These children need us to be there for them and let them tell us personal stories." Students were also able to relate this skill to interactions with others as well: "The importance of listening is a valuable skill that I can use in interpersonal relationships." After working with ten- to twelve-year-old children on expressing their feelings, one student affirmed, "I will definitely be a better listener especially if I don't know where people are coming from because I've learned everyone handles situations differently and just because something might not be a struggle for me, it could easily be a struggle for someone else."

## *Social Development*

Although the students were not asked to reflect on their personal feelings regarding community service, twenty-five percent of students reported that this service-learning experience positively influenced their feelings towards volunteering. Following their placements, students made comments such as: "As a result of my volunteering, I have learned that participating in such volunteer programs is beneficial. Volunteers are essential to the community, and without volunteers, those in need of support would be helpless." "Volunteering for an organization is well worth a person's time and energy." "I have learned the importance of volunteering, to become a part of the society and community." Others recommended that everyone should participate in community service. As one student declared, "I think that if everyone volunteered at some point in their lives, they would feel better about themselves." Another student, who spent her service-learning hours with a program aimed at keeping students in school, supported this idea by stating: "I think it should be a requirement for everyone to give up part of their time to donate to others who really need it."

Additionally, students completing this brief service-learning experience felt more committed to participating in similar activities in the future. One student stated, "Performing community service is great for everyone involved. This experience has helped me see just how important my small contributions can be. I see myself performing more community service in the future." Another student who mentored a third grader through the Any Baby Can program vowed, "I will continue to volunteer to help children who need a little extra time with their homework."

## *Academic Development*

This brief service-learning experience also helped students process and synthesize the information they learned in the classroom. In fact, over sixty percent of the students reported a better understanding of the course content as a result of the service-learning experience. More specifically, one course objective was to acquire knowledge regarding the issues diverse families face. One student commented, "To actually hear and witness the emotions [children] go through due to unstable homes exceeds what I was only hearing from the lecture. I have used the lectures to handle uncomfortable situations I have found myself in. The lectures have helped me provide better guidance to each of the children I interacted with." Another student reported, "This experience really complemented with what we learned in class this semester. We studied the various family forms and the complications that arise with each family form. While talking to the kids, I asked about the family forms they came from. I was intrigued to notice the correlation between the behaviors of the children and their family form."

A student who was given the opportunity to work with many different nontraditional families in a parent/child education program stated,

"The [family diversity] class laid the foundation and the hands-on experience made it stick and give it more meaning." Another student commented, "I think being given the chance to relate learned topics to the actual children made this a very beneficial experience. I feel like I can sit in a classroom and learn information, but if I can observe what I'm learning, it makes more sense."

The assignment gave others actual experience with some of the specific concepts from the course: "A lot of things I witnessed during this experience complimented what we discussed in class lectures regarding foster care. Substitute and foster caregivers have ill-defined roles/norms and I actually felt a bit of that 'role ambiguity' from time to time." Another student reported that after discussing the various family forms in class, she was able to recognize the positives, as well as the negatives, of parents who have been separated, single working moms, and grandparents raising their grandkids. Another student stated, "In class we talked about the loyalty conflicts [foster] children face. I realized during this experience that the children do face this issue. Many of the foster children will not give up their loyalty to their parents and this sometimes results in bitterness and lack of appreciation for their foster parents."

A student who had been involved in a parent education program stated, "I am a very hands-on learner and I need to experience things to be able to fully understand the concept. During the program, I was able to connect information from the classroom with what I was experiencing with the families; therefore, I was able to better understand the information." One student simply said, "I was able to use what I've learned in class in my interactions with children and their families. [However,] some things are better learned through hands-on experience." Another student was able to integrate the things she had learned from several courses: "I'm a firm believer in learning through experience. This experience has let me put to use not only what I've learned in this class, but also my other classes. This class has taught me to recognize different family forms and to be more tolerant of them. My other classes have taught me to look for developmental delays, attachment issues, and what is developmentally appropriate for children."

Additionally, about 30 percent of the students believed they learned more through their service-learning than in the actual classroom. After working at a local high school with teenage mothers, one student expressed, "I think learning through experience has significantly taught me more than learning in the classroom. It's very different when you actually see the family forms interact and they become real instead of a statistic on paper." After mentoring a fifteen year old with a criminal record, one student reported, "I have always learned best through hands-on experiences. I think it's great to learn material in class to give you prior knowledge and then having the opportunity to go out and use it is essential to active learning. Experience teaches you things you can't learn in class lectures. You're faced with real issues, not just research." Another student who worked with ten to twelve year olds while their parents attended a parent education class stated, "For me personally, learning through experience has taught me more because of the interaction with people. The information I've learned in class helped me through my volunteer experience because I knew what to expect to a certain extent." Lastly, one student reported, "You can only learn so much from a book and a teacher, but in real life situations, you understand and see the feelings and emotions firsthand. I have learned more being in the field than in the classroom. It was an experience I suggest everyone have because it opened my eyes, my mind, and my heart."

## *DISCUSSION*

Consistent with previous research, the students' reflections demonstrated the benefits of integrating service-learning into a family science course, even when the experience was brief (15 hours). They learned numerous valuable lessons about themselves and their future careers. Moreover, they became more accepting of others and they realized the importance of service to one's community. Students who engaged in service-learning were able to process and synthesize the information they learned in the classroom by experiencing course content in a real-world setting. As Eby (2001) noted, service-learning "has promise to enrich Family Science courses and the Family Science curriculum by helping students learn at deep levels through interaction with real community issues" (p. 10).

This study also makes a distinctive contribution to the literature because it is one of the few to examine the personal, professional, interpersonal, social, and academic development of students who complete a brief service-learning assignment as part of a family science course. By examining all areas of student development, a more comprehensive view of the experience is provided. At the same time, however, the results of this study must be interpreted with some caution because of methodological limitations.

First, an experimental design was not employed; thus, we are unable to determine the impact that extraneous variables (i.e., maturation, history, etc.) may have had on our findings. Ideally, future research should utilize a control group to determine the effect that service-learning has on student development. Furthermore, longitudinal studies that examine the students' personal, professional, interpersonal, social, and academic development should be conducted to assess both the short-term and long-term impact service-learning has on student development. In addition, "a pre-post design would allow researchers to evaluate student learning [and development] as a process" (Walker et al., 2003, p. 2).

Second, because the data were based on self-report, social desirability bias may be a potential limitation. Although the professor attempted to decrease this bias by instructing students to report both positive and negative experiences, the students tended to report unusually favorable outcomes. This finding is consistent with previous research on service-learning outcomes in family science courses (Karasik & Berke, 2001; Walker et al., 2003); however, future studies could expand upon self-report by including the perspectives of the service-learning site supervisors as well as the individuals and families served by the students. In addition, standardized measures could be employed in order to quantitatively examine student learning and development over the course of the semester.

Lastly, because the sample was homogeneous in nature (i.e., all female, drawn from one class, etc.), our study lacks generalizability. Additionally, it has been found that students' interest in the subject matter influences how much service-learning enhances their development (Astin et al., 2001). Therefore, because the students were mainly family and child development majors, who are likely to be interested in the course material to begin with, they also may have been inclined to report greater benefits from the service-learning experience. Thus, more diverse populations should be used to determine the impact that service-learning has on the development of students from a wide range of backgrounds.

Although there are notable limitations in this study, the findings yield some salient implications for curriculum development. First, when following a few fundamental guidelines (see Bringle & Hatcher, 2004; Eby, 2001; and Galbraith, 2002 for a complete overview of best practices), service-learning can be an effective pedagogical tool for teaching family science courses. Specifically, when integrating service-learning into their family science courses, it is suggested that faculty members adhere to the following guidelines.

1. Provide a list of potential sites where students may complete their service-learning hours. The sites should provide students with a high level of responsibility, direct contact with children and/or families, and opportunities to integrate course content (Eyler & Giles, 1999). However, students should have the option of choosing an equally appropriate site.
2. If students are allowed to choose alternative sites, establish specific criteria for selecting sites (i.e., must have direct contact with children and/or families, must be related to course objectives, etc.) and require students to have their sites pre-approved by their professor.
3. Encourage students to interact with individuals from diverse backgrounds.
4. Articulate clear objectives for both the student and the site supervisor.
5. Consistently integrate course content and service-learning experiences (Eby, 2001).
6. Provide opportunities for students to reflect, share their service-learning experiences, and discuss how their experiences relate to the course content (Eby, 2001; Eyler & Giles, 1999; Galbraith, 2002; Terry & Bohnenberger, 2003). This can be done through a variety of ways including journaling, reflection papers, small group discussion, class presentations, and so forth.

Furthermore, in addition to the academic advantages of service-learning, the personal, interpersonal, and social benefits of service-learning are immeasurable. This is particularly relevant to the field of family science because these are essential qualities students must possess when working with individuals and families. Lastly, even when faculty members are pressed for time, the findings from this study demonstrate the benefits of incorporating brief service-learning experiences into the curriculum.

## REFERENCES

Astin, A. W. & Sax, L. J. (1998). How undergraduates are affected by service participation. *Journal of College Student Development, 39*, 251-263.

Astin, A. W., Vogelgesang, L. J., Ikeda, E. K., & Yee, J. K. (2001). *How service-learning affects students: Executive summary.* Los Angeles: Higher Education Research Institute, UCLA.

Berg, B. L. (1998). *Qualitative research methods for the social sciences (3rd ed.)*. Boston, MA: Allyn and Bacon.

Bringle, R. G. & Hatcher, J. A. (2004). Implementing service learning in higher education. *The Journal of Higher Education, 67*, 221-239.

Burnett, J. A., Hamel, D., & Long, L. (2004). Service-learning in graduate counselor education: Developing multicultural counseling competency. *Multicultural Counseling and Development, 32*, 180-191.

Conrad, D. & Hedin, D. (1982). The impact of experiential education on adolescent development. *Child & Youth Services, 4*, 57-76.

Crowner, D. (1992). The effects of service-learning on student participants. Paper presented at The National Society for Experiential Education, Newport, RI.

Dudderar, D. & Stover, L. T. (2003). Putting service-learning experiences at the heart of a teacher education curriculum. *Educational Research Quarterly, 27*, 18-32.

Eby, J. W. (2001). The promise of service-learning for family science: An overview. *Journal of Teaching in Marriage and Family, 1*, 1-13.

Eyler, J. & Giles, D. E. (1999). *Where's the learning in service-learning?* San Francisco: Jossey-Bass.

Galbraith, K. A. (2002). Integrating service-learning into human service and family science curriculum. *Journal of Teaching in Marriage and Family, 2*, 363-395.

Giles, D. E. & Eyler, J. (1994). The impact of a college community service laboratory on students' personal, social, and cognitive outcomes. *Journal of Adolescence, 17*, 327-339.

Hamilton, S. F. & Fenzel, L. M. (1988). The impact of volunteer experience on adolescent social development: Evidence of program effects. *Journal of Adolescent Research, 3*, 65-80.

Karasik, R. J. & Berke, D. L. (2001). Classroom and community: Experiential education in family studies and gerontology. *Journal of Teaching in Marriage and Family, 1*, 13-38.

Markus, G., Arbor, A., Howard, J. P. E., & King, D. C. (1993). Integrating community service and classroom instruction enhances learning: Results from an experiment. *Education Evaluation & Policy Analysis, 15*, 410-419.

Martin, A. (2001). The many faces of engagement, learning goals, and the principles of good practice in service-learning. *Journal of Family and Consumer Sciences Education, 19*, 38-40.

Morgan, W. (1997-1998). *Evaluation of school-based service-learning in Indiana*. Report prepared for Indiana Department of Education.

Morgan, W. & Streb, M. (2001). Building citizenship: How student voice in service develops civic values. *Social Science Quarterly, 82*, 155-169.

Scales, P. C., Blyth, D. A., Berkas, T. H., & Kielsmeier, J. C. (2000). The effects of service-learning on middle school students' social responsibility and academic success. *Journal of Early Adolescence, 20*, 332-358.

Sedlak, C. A., Doheny, M. O., Panthofer, N., & Anaya, E. (2003). Critical thinking in students' service-learning experiences. *College Teaching, 51*, 99-103.

Stukas, A. A., Clary, G. E., & Snyder, M. (1999). Service-learning: Who benefits and why. *Social Policy Report, 8*, 1-22.

Terry, A. W. & Bohnenberger, J. E. (2003). Service-learning: Fostering a cycle of caring in our gifted youth. *The Journal of Secondary Gifted Education, 15*, 23-32.

Walker, K., Blankemeyer, M., Richardson, R. A., & Kraynak, A. R. (2003). *Student reflections of service-learning in parenting education.* Poster presented at the annual meeting of the National Council on Family Relations, Vancouver, BC.

Yates, M. & Youniss, J. (1996). A developmental perspective on community service in adolescence. *Social Development, 5*, 85-111.

# Index

Academic development considerations, 266-266,274-276
Action-taking processes, 252-256
Active learning, 9-10,216-217
Activities, 66-75,172-173,225-256
 for advocacy skills education, 66-75. *See also* Advocacy skills education
 behavioral, 255-256
 goal-related, 172-173
 interpersonal *vs.* intrapersonal, 255
 service-learning, 119-120. *See also* Service-learning perspectives
 values-related, 172
Adoption and Safe Families Act. *See* ASFA (Adoption and Safe Families Act) of 1997
Advocacy skills education, 62-78
 activities for, 66-75
  Cooperative Extension outreach initiatives and, 69-70
  in-house advocacy and, 71
  interaction styles and, 73-74
  internships, 68-71
  issues-related knowledge, 67-68
  legislative and regulatory decision-making processes, 68-71
  persuasion techniques, 74-75
  strategies for, 76
  target audience identification, 71-73
 advocacy definitions and, 65-66
 background perspectives of, 64-66
 CFLE credential and, 63-64,73-74
 future perspectives of, 76-77
 NCFR and, 63-66
 overviews and summaries of, 63-66
 reference resources for, 77-78
 Special Milk Amendment and, 68-71
Alpert, Lily T., 7-24
American Association of Marriage and Family Therapists, 187-188,199-200
American Counseling Association, 148-149
American Psychological Association. *See* APA (American Psychological Association)
*Amicus curiae* (friends and court) briefs, 7-24
Anderson, Elaine A., 63-78
Anderson, Stephen A., 225-242
APA (American Psychological Association), 148-149, 187-188
ASFA (Adoption and Safe Families Act) of 1997, 14,29-30, 34-35,38-39
Assignment-related considerations, 14-16,157-158
 cross-cultural perspective courses and, 157-158
 graded assignments, 14-16
Audience identification, 71-73

Background perspectives. *See also under individual topics*
 of family dynamics, 102-104, 116-119,134-136,147-149, 166-167

cross-cultural perspectives,
    147-149
curricula-related perspectives,
    134-136
family resource management
    (integrative approaches),
    166-167
father-daughter relationship
    courses, 102-104
parenting education, 116-119
of family law and family policy,
    8-12,26-29,48-50,64-66,
    78-80
    advocacy skills education, 64-66
    cooperative research teams,
        26-29
    marginalized family
        involvement issues, 78-80
    pedagogical approaches, 8-12
    student-specific perspectives,
        48-50
of teaching techniques, 186-189,
    206-209,226-228,244-245,
    264-267
    clinical training perspectives,
        186-189
    family diversity courses,
        264-267
    forgiveness process evaluations,
        244-245
    psychoeducational and
        preventive approaches,
        226-228
    small-group
        learning-hypothetical
        families approaches, 206-209
*Barkey v. Commonwealth of VA,
    Alexandria Department of
    Social Services* (1986), 31-39
Basic topics. *See* Overviews and
    summaries
Behavioral activities, 255-256
Berke, Debra L., 3-5
Blankemeyer, Maureen, 115-131
Braun, Bonnie, 63-78

Britner, Preston A., 7-24,225-242
Brown, Irene Q., 225-242
Browning, Scott, 185-203
Building capacity processes, 81-95

Cain, Colleen, 205-223
Capacity building processes, 81-95
Career plans clarification, 121-122
Case law. *See* Court cases
Cerny, Jennifer M., 263-280
CFLE (Certified Family Life Educator)
    credential, 63-64,73-74
Child Welfare Act. *See* CWA (Child
    Welfare Act) of 1980
CL (cooperative learning) approaches,
    25-45,207-209. *See also*
    Cooperative research teams
Clinical training perspectives, 185-203
    background perspectives of,
        186-189
    benefits of, 200-202
    ethical concerns, 199-200
    experiential techniques, 186
    future perspectives of, 202
    overviews and summaries of,
        185-186
    reference resources for, 202-203
    role-playing exercises and, 187-199
        American Association of
            Marriage and Family
            Therapists and, 187-188,
            199-200
        APA and, 187-188
        applications of, 188-189
        Creating Families protocol and,
            189-196
        Ethical Principles of
            Psychologists and Code of
            Ethics and, 187-188,199-200
    student-specific perspectives of,
        196-199
Coding structures and schema, 31-37
Collins, Jeanne S., 185-203

Conceptual frameworks, 117-119, 171-174
Contextual learning, 10
Cooperative Extension, 79-97. *See also under individual topics*
  advocacy skills education and, 69-70
  marginalized family involvement issues and, 79-97
  outreach initiatives of, 69-70
Cooperative learning approaches. *See CL (cooperative learning) approaches*
Cooperative research teams, 25-45
  ASFA of 1997 and, 29-30,34-35, 38-39
  background perspectives of, 26-29
  CL approaches and, 25-45
  components of, 28-29
  cooperative research experiences and, 29-34
    coding structures and schema and, 31-37
    GTM and, 31-37
    LEXIS/NEXIS roles in, 29-30
    orientations, 30-34
    team meeting roles in, 34-37
  court cases and, 26,31-39
    Barkey v. Commonwealth of VA, Alexandria Department of Social Services (1986), 31-39
    Malave v. Fairfax County Department of Social Services (1999), 39
    Moore v. the City of East Cleveland (1977), 26
    Richmond Department of Social Services v. L.P. (2001), 38-39
  CWA of 1980 and, 34-35
  foster care perspectives of, 25-45
  future perspectives of, 42
  objectives for, 28-29
  outcomes for, 37-42
    faculty, 41-42
    graduate, 41
    undergraduate, 39-40
    overviews and summaries of, 25-26
    reference resources for, 43-45
Coran, Justin, 205-223
Course content and design-related concepts, 105-108,149-158
Court cases, 13-14,26,31-39
  Barkey v. Commonwealth of VA, Alexandria Department of Social Services (1986), 31-39
  DeShaney v. Winnebago County Social Services Department (1989), 13-14
  Malave v. Fairfax County Department of Social Services (1999), 39
  Moore v. the City of East Cleveland (1977), 26
  Richmond Department of Social Services v. L.P. (2001), 38-39
Craft of teaching family studies (strategies and tools). *See also under individual topics*
  background perspectives. *See Background perspectives*
  family dynamics, 99-183
    family resource management (integrative approaches), 165-182
    father-daughter relationship courses, 101-113
    international family education (cross-cultural perspectives), 147-164
    international family education (curricula-related perspectives), 133-145
    parenting education, 115-131
  family law and family policy, 7-98
    advocacy skills education, 63-78
    cooperative research teams, 25-45
    marginalized family involvement issues, 79-97
    pedagogical approaches, 7-24

student-specific perspectives,
47-62
future perspectives. *See* Future
perspectives
overviews and summaries, 3-5. *See
also* Overviews and
summaries
reference resources. *See* Reference
resources
service-learning perspectives,
115-131
family diversity courses,
263-280
parenting education, 115-131
teaching techniques, 193-280
clinical training perspectives,
185-203
family diversity courses,
263-280
forgiveness process evaluations,
243-261
psychoeducational and
preventive approaches,
225-242
small-group
learning-hypothetical
families approaches, 205-223
Creating Families protocol, 189-196
Creativity issues, 216-217
Credentialing considerations, 63-64,
73-74
Crisis intervention resource persons,
247
Critical thinking, 9-10
Cross-cultural perspectives, 147-164.
*See also* International family
education
American Counseling Association
and, 148-149
APA and, 148-149
background perspectives of,
147-149
course content and, 151-156
course development considerations
and, 149-158

course evaluations and, 158-160
course objectives and, 149-150
future perspectives of, 160
International Association of
Couples and Family
Counselors and, 148-149
overviews and summaries of,
147-148
projects and assignments and,
157-158
reference resources for, 160-162
student-specific perspectives and,
158-160
textbook considerations and,
156-157
Curricula-related perspectives
(international family
education), 133-145. *See also*
International family
education
background perspectives of,
134-136
future perspectives of, 143-144
overviews and summaries of,
133-136
reference resources for, 144-145
studies of, 136-142
textbook perspectives, 142-144
CWA (Child Welfare Act) of 1980,
34-35


Daughter-father relationship courses,
101-113
background perspectives of,
102-104
design of, 105-108
format, 105-106
grading, 105-106
interviews, 106
media and Web sites, 106
objectives, 105
reading assignments, 105-106
self-assignment quizzes, 108
future perspectives of, 111

overviews and summaries of, 101-113
positive relationships, 103-104
  benefits of, 104
  *vs.* negative relationships, 103-104
  unhappy marriages and divorce effects and, 104
reference resources for, 111-113
studies of, 108-111
  methods, 108-111
  results, 110
  samples, 108-111
Davison, Diane, 243-261
Decision-making processes, 68-71
Department of Health and Human Services. *See* DHHS (Department of Health and Human Services)
*DeShaney v. Winnebago County Social Services Department* (1989), 13-14
Design-related concepts, 105-108
Developmental assets frameworks, 121
DHHS (Department of Health and Human Services), 227
Disclosure, 254
Diversity (family) courses, 263-280. *See also* Service-learning perspectives
  academic development and, 266-267,274-276
  background perspectives of, 264-267
  future perspectives of, 277-278
  guidelines for, 277-278
  interpersonal development and, 265-266,271-273
  overviews and summaries of, 263-264
  personal development and, 264-265,268-271
  professional development and, 265,271
  reference resources for, 278-280

social development and, 266, 273-274
studies of, 264-278
Divorce-related impacts, 104
Dynamics, family, 99-183. *See also under individual topics*
family resource management (integrative approaches), 165-182
father-daughter relationship courses, 101-113
international family education (cross-cultural perspectives), 147-164

Emotional wound healing processes, 247-252
Ethical concerns, 199-200
Ethical Principles of Psychologists and Code of Ethics, 187-188, 199-200
Evaluation-related considerations, 11-12,17-20,158-160, 213-214,235-237. *See also under individual topics*
  course evaluations (general), 11-12
  cross-cultural perspective courses and, 158-160
  psychoeducational and preventive approaches and, 235-237
  small-group learning-hypothetical families approaches and, 213-214
  teaching evaluations, 17-20
Experiential clinical training techniques, 186. *See also* Clinical training perspectives

*Families in Eastern Europe* (Robila), 143
*Families in Global Perspective* (Roopnarine, J. and Gielen, U.), 143

Family diversity courses, 263-280. *See also* Service-learning perspectives
  academic development and, 266-267, 274-276
  background perspectives of, 264-267
  future perspectives of, 277-278
  guidelines for, 277-278
  interpersonal development and, 265-266, 271-273
  overviews and summaries of, 263-264
  pedagogical approaches and, 7-24. *See also* Pedagogical approaches
  personal development and, 264-265, 268-271
  professional development and, 265, 271
  reference resources for, 278-280
  social development and, 266, 273-274
  studies of, 264-278
Family dynamics, 99-183. *See also under individual topics*
  family resource management (integrative approaches), 165-182
  father-daughter relationship courses, 101-113
  international family education, 133-164
    cross-cultural perspectives, 147-164
    curricula-related perspectives, 133-145
  parenting education, 115-131
Family group construction processes, 209-210, 221-222
*Family in Global Perspectives: A Gendered Journey, The* (Leeder, E.), 143
Family law and family policy, 7-98. *See also under individual topics*
  advocacy skills education, 63-78
  cooperative research teams, 25-45
  marginalized family involvement issues, 79-97
  pedagogical approaches, 7-24
  student-specific perspectives, 47-62
Family resource management (integrative approaches), 165-182
  background perspectives of, 166-167
  course descriptions for, 168-181
    conceptual frameworks, 171-174
    goals activities, 173
    Gross et al. model, 168-171
    management processes, 176-179
    management system inputs, 174-176
    new model, 168-171
    objectives, 168-169
    outcomes, 179-181
    problem-solving case studies, 171
    values activities, 172
  future perspectives of, 181
  NCFR and, 165-167
  need for, 167
  overviews and summaries of, 165-167
  reference resources for, 181-182
  *Resource Management for Individuals and Families* (Goldsmith) and, 167
  *Solution, The* (Mellin) and, 178
Family studies teaching concepts (strategies and tools). *See also under individual topics*
  background perspectives. *See* Background perspectives
  family dynamics, 99-183
    family resource management (integrative approaches), 165-182
    father-daughter relationship courses, 101-113

## Index

international family education
(cross-cultural perspectives),
147-164
international family education
(curricula-related
perspectives), 133-145
parenting education, 115-131
family law and family policy, 7-98
advocacy skills education, 63-78
cooperative research teams,
25-45
marginalized family
involvement issues, 79-97
pedagogical approaches, 7-24
student-specific perspectives,
47-62
future perspectives. *See* Future
perspectives
overviews and summaries, 3-5. *See
also* Overviews and
summaries
reference resources. *See* Reference
resources
service-learning perspectives,
115-131
family diversity courses,
263-280
parenting education, 115-131
teaching techniques, 193-280
clinical training perspectives,
185-203
family diversity courses,
263-280
forgiveness process evaluations,
243-261
psychoeducational and
preventive approaches,
225-242
small-group
learning-hypothetical
families approaches, 205-223
Family Violence Initiative. *See* FVI
(Family Violence Initiative)
Father-daughter relationship courses,
101-113

background perspectives of,
102-104
design of, 105-108
format, 105-106
grading, 105-106
interviews, 106-108
media and Web sites, 106
objectives, 105
reading assignments, 105-106
self-assignment quizzes, 108
future perspectives of, 111
overviews and summaries of,
101-113
positive relationships, 103-104
benefits of, 104
*vs.* negative relationships,
103-104
unhappy marriages and divorce
effects and, 104
reference resources for, 111-113
studies of, 108-111
methods, 108-111
results, 110
samples, 108-111
Feedback, quantitative *vs.* qualitative,
17
Forgiveness process evaluations,
243-261
action-taking processes and,
252-256
background perspectives of,
244-245
behavioral activities and, 255-256
crisis intervention resource persons
and, 247
disclosure and, 254
emotional impacts and, 254-255
emotional wound healing processes
and, 247-252
forgiveness interventions and,
256-257
future perspectives of, 259-260
group participation and, 254
interpersonal *vs.* intrapersonal
activities, 255

leader modeling and, 254
need for, 245
overviews and summaries of,
 243-245
reference resources for, 260-261
in workshop and classroom settings,
 243-261
 classroom settings, 256-257
 workshop settings, 245-256
Format-related concepts, 105-106
Foster care perspectives, 25-45
Frameworks, conceptual, 117-119,
 171-174
Friends and court *(amicus curiae)*
 briefs, 7-24
Fundamental topics. *See* Overviews
 and summaries
Future career plans clarification,
 121-122
Future perspectives. *See also under*
 *individual topics*
 of family dynamics, 111,129-130,
 143-144,160,181
 cross-cultural perspectives, 160
 curricula-related perspectives,
 143-144
 family resource management
  (integrative approaches), 181
 father-daughter relationship
  courses, 111
 parenting education, 129-130
 of family law and family policy,
 20-21,42,76-77,93-95
 advocacy skills education, 76-77
 cooperative research teams, 42
 marginalized family
  involvement issues, 93-95
 pedagogical approaches, 20-21
 of teaching techniques, 202,
 218-220,239-240,259-260,
 277-278
 clinical training perspectives,
 202
 family diversity courses,
 277-278

forgiveness process evaluations,
 259-260
psychoeducational and
 preventive approaches,
 239-240
small-group
 learning-hypothetical
 families approaches, 218-220
FVI (Family Violence Initiative),
 229-240

Goals activities, 173
Grading-related considerations, 14-16,
 105-106,213-214
Greder, Kimberly, 79-97
Gross et al. model, 168-171
Grounded Theory Method. *See* GTM
 (Grounded Theory Method)
Group work insights, 121
GTM (Grounded Theory Method),
 31-37

Healing processes, emotional wounds,
 247-252
Henderson, Tammy L., 25-45
Hilton, Jeanne M., 165-182
Historical perspectives. *See*
 Background perspectives
Holgerson, Kathleen, 225-242
Hypothetical families-small group
 learning approaches, 205-223
 active learning and, 216-217
 applications of, 215-220
 background perspectives of,
 206-209
 cautions for, 217-219
 CL approaches and, 207-209. *See*
  *also* CL (cooperative
  learning) approaches
 creativity issues and, 216-217
 evaluations of, 213-214
 examples for, 221-223

family group construction
   processes, 209-210, 221-222
 future perspectives of, 218-220
 grading considerations for,
   213-214
 in-class procedures for, 212-213
 methods for, 209-215
 objectives of, 207-209
 online supplements for, 214-215
 overviews and summaries of,
   205-207
 reference resources for, 220
 scenario considerations for,
   210-212, 222-223
 success of, 215-216

In-class procedures, 212-213
In-house advocacy, 71. *See also*
   Advocacy skills education
Instructor recommendations, 60-61
Integrative approaches (family
      resource management),
      165-182
 background perspectives of,
   166-167
 course descriptions for, 168-181
   conceptual frameworks, 171-174
   goals activities, 173
   Gross et al. model, 168-171
   management processes, 176-179
   management system inputs,
      174-176
   new model, 168-171
   objectives, 168-169
   outcomes, 179-181
   problem-solving case studies,
      171
   values activities, 172
 future perspectives of, 181
 NCFR and, 165-167
 need for, 167
 overviews and summaries of,
   165-167
 reference resources for, 181-182

*Resource Management for*
   *Individuals and Families*
   (Goldsmith) and, 167
 *Solution, The* (Mellin) and, 178
Interaction styles, 73-74
International Association of Couples
   and Family Counselors,
   148-149
International family education,
   147-164. *See also under*
   *individual topics*
 cross-cultural perspectives, 147-164
   American Counseling
      Association and, 148-149
   APA and, 148-149
   background perspectives of,
      147-149
   course content and, 151-156
   course development
      considerations and, 149-158
   course evaluations and, 158-160
   course objectives and, 149-150
   future perspectives of, 160
   International Association of
      Couples and Family
      Counselors and, 148-149
   overviews and summaries of,
      147-148
   projects and assignments and,
      157-158
   reference resources for, 160-162
   student-specific perspectives
      and, 158-160
   textbook considerations and,
      156-157
 curricula-related perspectives,
      133-145
   background perspectives of,
      134-136
   future perspectives of, 143-144
   overviews and summaries of,
      133-136
   reference resources for, 144-145
   studies of, 136-142

textbook considerations,
142-144
*International Perspectives on Family Violence and Abuse: A Cognitive Ecological Approach* (Malley-Morrison), 143-144
Interpersonal issues, 255,265-266, 271-273
Intervention-related considerations, 230-231,256-257
Interviews, 106
Intrapersonal issues, 120
Introductory topics. *See* Overviews and summaries
Issues-related knowledge, 67-68

Kopera-Frye, Karen, 165-182
Koropeckyj-Cox, Tanya, 205-223
Kraynak, Audrey, 115-131

Large introductory courses, 205-223. *See also* Small-group learning-hypothetical families approaches
Law and policy (family) concepts, 7-98
 advocacy skills education, 63-78
 cooperative research teams, 25-45
 marginalized family involvement issues, 79-97
 pedagogical approaches, 7-24
 student-specific perspectives, 47-62
Leader modeling, 254
Legislative decision-making processes, 68-71
Leite, Randy, 47-62
LEXIS/NEXIS roles, 29-30
*Lives Across Cultures: Cross Cultural Human Development* (Mutter and Kosmitzki), 143
Logistical considerations, parenting education, 128-129. *See also* Parenting education

*Malave v. Fairfax County Department of Social Services* (1999), 39
Management-related issues, 165-182
 family resource management, 165-182. *See also* Family resource management (integrative approaches)
 management processes, 176-179
 management system inputs, 174-176
Marginalized family involvement issues, 79-97
 background perspectives of, 78-80
 capacity building processes, 81-95
 Cooperative Extension and, 79-97
 future perspectives of, 93-95
 overviews and summaries of, 79
 reference resources for, 95-96
 *ROWELL Poverty Simulation* and, 79-97
 *Sharing a Family's Story* and, 79-97
*Mate Selection Across Cultures* (Hamon and Ingoldsby), 144
McWey, Lenore, 25-45
Media-related considerations, 106
Medora, Nilufer P., 147-164
Models, family resource management, 168-171
*Moore v. the City of East Cleveland* (1977), 26
Motivation, 10
Mutchler, Matthew S., 243-261

National Council on Family Relations. *See* NCFR (National Council on Family Relations)
National Family Violence Survey, 227-228
NCFR (National Council on Family Relations), 63-66,165-167
Negative father-daughter relationships, 103-104
Nelson, Bryan, 185-203
Nielsen, Linda, 101-113

O'Neil, James M., 225-261
Online supplements, 214-215
Oral presentations, 16
Orientations, 30-34
Outcomes-related considerations, 17-20,37-42,179-181. *See also under individual topics*
   for cooperative research teams, 37-42
   for family resource management (integrative approaches), 179-181
   for pedagogical approaches, 17-20
Outreach initiatives, 69-70
Overviews and summaries. *See also under individual topics*
   of family dynamics, 115-117, 133-136,147-148,165-167
     cross-cultural perspectives, 147-148
     curricula-related perspectives, 133-136
     family resource management (integrative approaches), 165-167
     father-daughter relationship courses, 101-113
     parenting education, 115-117
   of family law and family policy, 7-8,25-26,47,63-66,79
     advocacy skills education, 63-66
     cooperative research teams, 25-26
     marginalized family involvement issues, 79
     pedagogical approaches, 7-8
     student-specific perspectives, 47
   of teaching techniques, 185-186, 205-207,225-245,263-264
     clinical training perspectives, 185-186
     family diversity courses, 263-264
     forgiveness process evaluations, 243-245
     psychoeducational and preventive approaches, 225-242
     small-group learning-hypothetical families approaches, 205-207

Parenting education, 115-131. *See also* Service-learning perspectives
   background perspectives of, 116-119
   conceptual frameworks for, 117-119
   future perspectives of, 129-130
   logistical considerations for, 128-129
   overviews and summaries of, 115-117
   parent evaluations of, 124-126
   reference resources for, 130-131
   roles of, 126-128
   as service-learning activities, 119-120
   student-specific perspectives of, 120-124
     concerns and fears, 121
     developmental assets frameworks and, 121
     education delivery impacts, 122-124
     future career plans clarification, 121-122
     group work insights, 121
     intrapersonal issues, 120
     self-knowledge impacts, 120-121
Pedagogical approaches, 7-24
   active learning, 9-10
   ASFA of 1997 and, 14
   background perspectives of, 8-12
   contextual learning, 10
   course application components and issues for, 11-20

    *amicus curiae* (friends and
        court) briefs, 7-24
    course descriptions, 13-20
    course evaluations, 11-12
    course objectives, 13-14
    graded assignments, 14-16
    oral presentations, 16
    outcomes, 17-20
    policy briefs, 15-16
    quantitative *vs.* qualitative
        feedback, 17
    research papers, 14
    teaching evaluations, 17-20
  critical thinking, 9-10
  *DeShaney v. Winnebago County
     Social Services Department*
     (1989) and, 13-14
  future perspectives of, 20-21
  motivation, 10
  overviews and summaries of, 7-8
  reference resources for, 21-23
  writing skills, 10-11
Personal development considerations,
    264-265, 268-271
Persuasion techniques, 74-75
Policy and law (family) concepts, 7-98
    advocacy skills education, 63-78
    cooperative research teams, 25-45
    marginalized family involvement
        issues, 79-97
    pedagogical approaches, 7-24
    student-specific perspectives, 47-62
Positive father-daughter relationships,
    103-104
Preparation processes, 229-230
Presentations, oral, 16
Preventive and psychoeducational
    approaches, 225-242
    background perspectives of,
        226-228
    future perspectives of, 239-240
    FVI and, 229-240
    importance of, 237-240
    intervention definitions for,
        230-231

National Family Violence Survey
    and, 227-228
overviews and summaries of,
    225-242
program preparation processes and,
    229-230
psychological abuse prevention
    contexts and, 228-242
reference resources for, 240-242
studies of, 229-240
Problem-solving case studies, 171,
    256-257
Process evaluations and forgiveness
    teaching, 243-261
    action-taking processes and,
        252-256
    background perspectives of,
        244-245
    behavioral activities and, 255-256
    crisis intervention resource persons
        and, 247
    disclosure and, 254
    emotional impacts and, 254-255
    emotional wound healing processes
        and, 247-252
    future perspectives of, 259-260
    interpersonal *vs.* intrapersonal
        activities, 255
    leader modeling and, 254
    need for, 245
    overviews and summaries of,
        243-245
    reference resources for, 260-261
    in workshop and classroom settings,
        243-261
    workshop settings, 245-256
Professional development
    considerations, 265, 271
Program preparation processes,
    229-230
Psychoeducational and preventive
    approaches, 225-242
    background perspectives of,
        226-228
    evaluations of, 235-237

future perspectives of, 239-240
FVI and, 229-240
importance of, 237-240
intervention definitions for,
 230-231
National Family Violence Survey
 and, 227-228
overviews and summaries of,
 225-242
program preparation processes and,
 229-230
psychological abuse prevention
 contexts and, 228-242
reference resources for, 240-242
studies of, 229-240
Psychological abuse prevention
 contexts, 228-242


Quantitative *vs.* qualitative feedback, 17


Reading assignments, 105-106
Reference resources. *See also under
 individual topics*
 for family dynamics, 111-113,
  130-131,144-145,160-162,
  181-182
  cross-cultural perspectives,
   160-162
  curricula-related perspectives,
   144-145
  family resource management
   (integrative approaches),
   181-182
  father-daughter relationship
   courses, 111-113
  parenting education, 130-131
 for family law and family policy,
  21-23,43-45,61-62,77-78,
  95-96
  advocacy skills education, 77-78
  cooperative research teams,
   43-45

marginalized family
 involvement issues, 95-96
pedagogical approaches, 21-23
student-specific perspectives,
 61-62
for teaching techniques, 202-203,
 220,240-242,260-261,
 278-280
 clinical training perspectives,
  202-203
 family diversity courses,
  278-280
 forgiveness process evaluations,
  260-261
 psychoeducational and
  preventive approaches,
  240-242
 small-group
  learning-hypothetical
  families approaches, 220
Regulatory decision-making processes,
 68-71
Research papers, 14
Resource management, family,
 165-182. *See also* Family
 resource management
 (integrative approaches)
*Resource Management for Individuals
 and Families* (Goldsmith),
 167
Resources, reference. *See* Reference
 resources
Richardson, Rhonda A., 115-131
*Richmond Department of Social
 Services v. L.P.* (2001), 38-39
Robila, Mihaela, 133-145
Rohner, Ronald P., 225-242
Role-playing exercises, 185-203
 American Association of Marriage
  and Family Therapists and,
  187-188,199-200
 APA and, 187-188
 applications of, 188-189
 background perspectives of,
  186-189

benefits of, 187-188, 200-202
caveats for, 187-188
clinical training perspectives of, 185-203
Creating Families protocol and, 189-196
Ethical Principles of Psychologists and Code of Ethics (APA), 187-188, 199-200
experiential clinical training techniques, 186
future perspectives of, 202
overviews and summaries of, 185-186
reference resources for, 202-203
student-specific perspectives of, 196-199
*ROWELL Poverty Simulation,* 79-97

Scenario considerations, 210-212, 222-223
Schema, coding, 31-37
Selected readings. *See* Reference resources
Self-assignment quizzes, 108
Self-knowledge impacts, 120-121
Service-learning perspectives, 115-131
  family diversity courses, 263-280
    academic development and, 266-267, 274-276
    background perspectives of, 264-267
    future perspectives of, 277-278
    guidelines for, 277-278
    interpersonal development and, 265-266, 271-273
    overviews and summaries of, 263-264
    personal development and, 264-265, 268-271
    professional development and, 265, 271
    reference resources for, 278-280
    social development and, 266, 273-274
    studies of, 264-278
  parenting education, 115-131
    background perspectives of, 116-119
    conceptual frameworks for, 117-119
    future perspectives of, 129-130
    logistical considerations for, 128-129
    overviews and summaries of, 115-117
    parent evaluations of, 124-126
    reference resources for, 130-131
    roles of, 126-128
    as service-learning activities, 119-120
    student-specific perspectives of, 120-124
*Sharing a Family's Story,* 79-97
Small-group learning-hypothetical families approaches, 205-223
  active learning and, 216-217
  applications of, 215-220
  background perspectives of, 206-209
  cautions for, 217-219
  CL approaches and, 207-209. *See also* CL (cooperative learning) approaches
  creativity issues and, 216-217
  evaluations of, 213-214
  examples for, 221-223
  family group construction processes, 209-210, 221-222
  future perspectives of, 218-220
  grading considerations for, 213-214
  in-class procedures for, 212-213
  methods for, 209-215
  objectives of, 207-209
  online supplements for, 214-215
  overviews and summaries of, 205-207
  reference resources for, 220

scenario considerations for, 210-212, 222-223
success of, 215-216
Social development considerations, 266, 273-274
*Solution, The* (Mellin), 178
Special Milk Amendment, 68-71
Strategies and tools (family studies teaching concepts). *See also under individual topics*
background perspectives. *See* Background perspectives
family dynamics, 99-183
family resource management (integrative approaches), 165-182
father-daughter relationship courses, 101-113
international family education (cross-cultural perspectives), 147-164
international family education (curricula-related perspectives), 133-145
parenting education, 115-131
family law and family policy, 7-98
advocacy skills education, 63-78
cooperative research teams, 25-45
marginalized family involvement issues, 79-97
pedagogical approaches, 7-24
student-specific perspectives, 47-62
future perspectives. *See* Future perspectives
overviews and summaries, 3-5. *See also* Overviews and summaries
reference resources. *See* Reference resources
service-learning perspectives, 115-131
family diversity courses, 263-280
parenting education, 115-131

teaching techniques, 193-280
clinical training perspectives, 185-203
family diversity courses, 263-280
forgiveness process evaluations, 243-261
psychoeducational and preventive approaches, 225-242
small-group learning-hypothetical families approaches, 205-223
Structures, coding, 31-37
Student-specific perspectives, 47-62, 120-124, 158-160, 196-199. *See also under individual topics*
background perspectives of, 48-50
of clinical training perspectives, 196-199
of cross-cultural perspectives, 158-160
future perspectives of, 60-61
instructor recommendations and, 60-61
overviews and summaries of, 47
of parenting education, 120-124
reference resources for, 61-62
studies of, 50-61
discussions, 57-60
methods, 50-52
results, 52-57
Suggested readings. *See* Reference resources
Summary topics. *See* Overviews and summaries
System inputs, management, 174-176

Target audience identification, 71-73
Taylor, Alan C., 133-145
Teaching evaluations, 17-20
Teaching family studies concepts (strategies and tools). *See also under individual topics*

background perspectives. *See*
   Background perspectives
family dynamics, 99-183
   father-daughter relationship
     courses, 101-113
   international family education
     (cross-cultural perspectives),
     147-164
   international family education
     (curricula-related
     perspectives), 133-145
   parenting education, 115-131
family law and family policy, 7-98
   advocacy skills education, 63-78
   cooperative research teams,
     25-45
   marginalized family
     involvement issues, 79-97
   pedagogical approaches, 7-24
   student-specific perspectives,
     47-62
future perspectives. *See* Future
   perspectives
overviews and summaries, 3-5. *See
   also* Overviews and
   summaries
reference resources. *See* Reference
   resources
service-learning perspectives,
   115-131,263-280
   family diversity courses,
     263-280
   parenting education, 115-131
teaching techniques, 193-280
   clinical training perspectives,
     185-203
   family diversity courses, 263-280
   forgiveness process evaluations,
     243-261
   psychoeducational and
     preventive approaches,
     225-242
   small-group
     learning-hypothetical
     families approaches, 205-223

Teaching techniques, 193-280
   clinical training perspectives,
     185-203
   family diversity courses, 263-280
   forgiveness teaching, 243-261. *See
     also* Forgiveness process
     evaluations
   psychoeducational and preventive
     approaches, 225-242
   small-group learning-hypothetical
     families approaches, 205-223
Textbook-related considerations,
   142-144,156-157
   for cross-cultural perspectives,
     156-157
   for curricula-related perspectives,
     142-144
Toews, Michelle, 263-280
Tools and strategies (family studies
   teaching concepts). *See also
   under individual topics*
   background perspectives. *See*
     Background perspectives
   family dynamics, 99-183
     family resource management
       (integrative approaches),
       165-182
     father-daughter relationship
       courses, 101-113
     international family education
       (cross-cultural perspectives),
       147-164
     international family education
       (curricula-related
       perspectives), 133-145
     parenting education, 115-131
   family law and family policy, 7-98
     advocacy skills education, 63-78
     cooperative research teams,
       25-45
     marginalized family
       involvement issues, 79-97
     pedagogical approaches, 7-24
     student-specific perspectives,
       47-62

future perspectives. *See* Future
perspectives
overviews and summaries, 3-5. *See also* Overviews and summaries
reference resources. *See* Reference resources
service-learning perspectives, 115-131
  family diversity courses, 263-280
  parenting education, 115-131
teaching techniques, 193-280
  clinical training perspectives, 185-203
  family diversity courses, 263-280
  forgiveness process evaluations, 243-261
  psychoeducational and preventive approaches, 225-242
  small-group learning-hypothetical families approaches, 205-223
Trachtenberg, Jennifer, 243-261

Unhappy marriage-related impacts, 104

Values activities, 172
Viramontez Anguiano, Ruben P., 47-62

Walker, Kathleen A., 115-131
Walker, Susan K., 63-78
Warning, Jeanne, 79-97
Web site issues, 106
Wisensale, Steven K., 3-5
Workshop settings, forgiveness teaching, 243-261. *See also* Forgiveness process evaluations
Wound healing processes, emotional, 247-252
Writing skills, 10-11